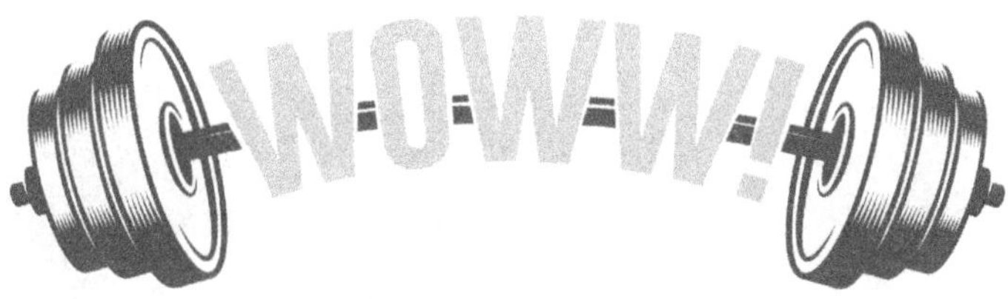

I *CAN* LOSE WEIGHT!

Don't wish for it

Work
On
Wellness
Wish

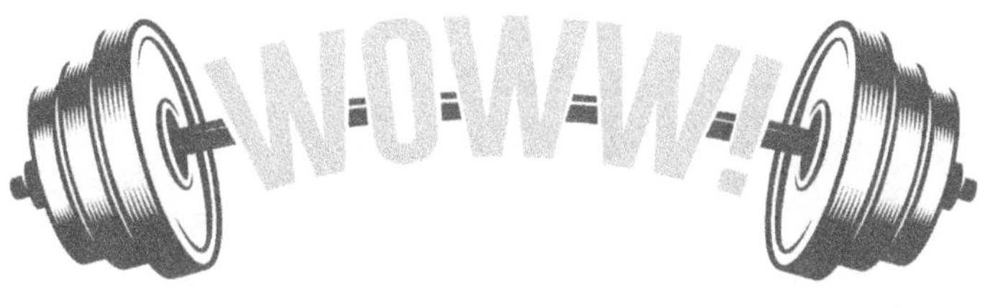

I *CAN* LOSE WEIGHT!

Essential Tools for a Lifestyle of Wellness

PIA FITZGERALD

The Wellness Tactician

XULON PRESS

Xulon Press
2301 Lucien Way #415
Maitland, FL 32751
407.339.4217
www.xulonpress.com

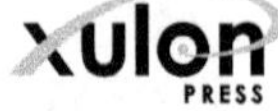

Printed in the United States of America.

ISBN-13: 978-1-54565-537-5

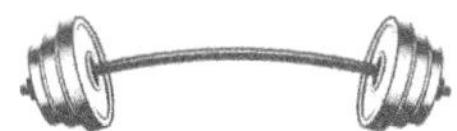

ACKNOWLEDGMENTS

Frank and Marcia Jarrett:
Thank you for cultivating the gifts of education and good health inside me. You two were the perfect vessels for one Pia Fitzgerald ☺.

Craig Lamont:
The best hubby ever! I enjoy being the wife on Team Fitzgerald.

Jessica and Khary:
You two are wonderful children with great things to offer the world. Keep exploring and living courageously.

Ariana:
Grandma loves you and cannot wait to share your books with the world.

Thank you to all my family, friends, clients, leaders, etc. **If you poured something into me, I am truly grateful.**

Love you all!
Pia Fitzgerald

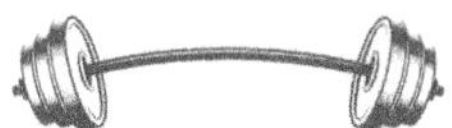

TABLE OF CONTENTS

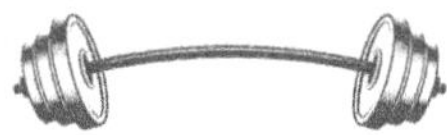

INSPIRATION FOR BOOK

"I WISH I could be fit and healthy while remaining overworked and overscheduled."

I used to believe the lie: Wish for something hard enough without doing the WORK required, and your wish will manifest. I dismissed the truth that some beliefs and habits would have to go as part of the WORK required to achieve my weight loss wellness goal. I believed this lie daily while pursuing a career and devoting 60-plus hours per week of my precious blood, sweat and tears. This lie led me to my highest weight ever of 197lbs! The funny thing is that I BELIEVED I could lose the weight and keep it off while stressing myself over matters that REALLY DID NOT MATTER.

What truly mattered was being a visual example of peace, joy, happiness, and prosperity. I NO LONGER desired to look like I took medication. I wanted to look, feel, and live the way I was created to be. Anything less would no longer be tolerated. I stopped WISHING I was fit and healthy and did the WORK required to achieve the state of health I desired and deserved.

This book is a GIFT to those who are riding the roller coaster of weight loss and desire to come off and enjoy a different, smoother ride in life. It is for those who want to ride the permanent lifestyle of wellness and embrace all the treasures that come along with it. It is for the person ready to WOWW! themselves and successfully WORK ON their WELLNESS WISH, lose weight and live out their WOWW!Factor!

WOWW! Work On your Wellness Wish
And lose weight!

Freedom Key—Say the following out loud
at least 3 times with energy:

WOWW! I CAN Lose Weight!

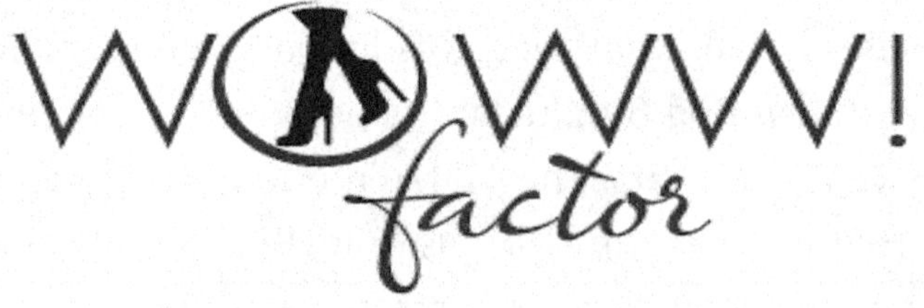

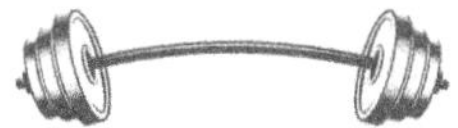

THE WOWW!FACTOR POWER TOOLS OF WELLNESS™

Below is a glimpse of the power tools you will use to achieve your WOWW!Factor.

WOWW! Tool—Priorities—The LOUDEST will drive your priorities. Make sure what you feast on emotionally, mentally, physically, spiritually, and relationally speak a language that pushes you towards achieving your WOWW!Factor and is not poisonous to your progress.

WOWW! Tool—Price—Investing in yourself is a must to yield a high return on investment and is necessary for achieving your WOWW!Factor.

WOWW! Tool—Perspective—Your vision determines your success. Your heart must see your WOWW!Factor in order to produce the actions that will help you achieve it.

WOWW! Tool—Permission—Sometimes we don't achieve our WOWW!Factor simply because we haven't given ourselves permission to be successful. Some of the most arresting obstacles to success are the ones we erect and hold ourselves hostage to…fear and doubt.

WOWW! Tool —Pause—Pausing is an essential discipline for achieving your WOWW!Factor and living a lifestyle of total wellness. A moment of stillness can open the door to new insight and ultimate abundance and a life of WOWW! I CAN Lose Weight!

WOWW! Tool—Process—To everything there is a process, even if it is not evident. Achieving your WOWW!Factor requires going through a collection of mini-processes that ultimately blend into one that yields sustainable SUCCESS.

Pick up the ***WOWW! I CAN Lose Weight Companion Guide*** (Ready Publications) for structured small group study material, additional resources, and *bonus* power tools of wellness. Join the online ***WOWW!Factor Experience*** at www.wowwfactorwomen.com for even MORE resources to help you lose weight and achieve that WOWW!Factor.

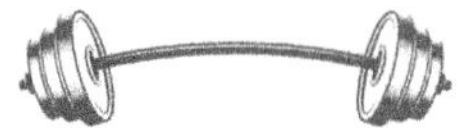

RULES OF ENGAGEMENT

The following segments infused throughout the text provide supplemental information and opportunities to APPLY the concepts in the book. **DO all of them**.

Wellness Red Flags alert you to common traps people experience when it comes to certain areas of wellness. Understanding the trap and its warning signal will allow you to be proactive while journeying to a lifestyle of total wellness.

Up Close and Personals are inspirational testimonies designed to remind you that you are not alone. It always helps to know someone else has traveled down a road that seems untrodden and lonely.

Freedom Keys provide an immediate activation to help create the neuropathway necessary for future wellness success. Do not skim through these keys.

WOWW! Recaps— are designed for reflection and activation of the concepts learned for that Power Tool. They are included at the end of each **Power Tool** section. Do not skip this process.

- **Wellness Declarations** are statements you vocalize as often as needed to activate the necessary internal shift. What comes out of your mouth has the power to create life or cause death! **Your words CAN move mountains!**

- **WOWW! *PROCESS* Power Tool of Wellness** requires you to complete a **start, stop,** and **keep** activation designed to apply the principles outlined in the section. Complete this portion in the journal section**.** USING the tools and embracing the principles WILL help you achieve your WOWW!Factor.

- **Reflections Pages** are included at the end of each section for **journaling.** *Journaling is essential for Working On your Wellness Wish.*

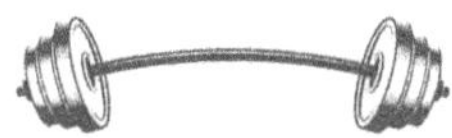

ACHIEVING YOUR WOWW!FACTOR PROTOCOL

How to best work on your wellness wishes with this book and win!

1. Schedule your reading time and HONOR it as an IMPORTANT appointment that cannot be canceled.

___

___

___

___

2. Reward yourself when you keep your appointment (use something other than food).

___

___

___

___

3. Create a visual map or use our suggested sample to illustrate your progress by consistently reading the book and honoring your reading appointments.

___

___

___

___

4. Use the **Reflection Section** for completing various activities and journaling about your WOWW! journey.

___

___

___

___

Journaling is an essential discipline of wellness. You don't have to write a dissertation each day, and there is no need to fret over spelling or punctuation. This is for YOUR EYES AND HEART only! There may be days you only record 3 words. Establishing a daily habit of journaling will help develop the discipline necessary for activating your WOWW!Factor and losing weight for good.

5. Enlist an accountability partner or a group of like-minded folks with the same goal to lose weight. **Identify 3 potential accountability partners for your WOWW!Factor.** Read and discuss the book together. (Purchase the ***WOWW! I CAN Lose Weight Companion Guide*** for more tools and guidelines.)

____

____

____

____

6. Release the desire for a quick fix; it's temporary. Opt for total transformation.

____

____

____

____

7. Get the *WOWW!Factor Companion Guide*. It contains lots of supplemental material that you can benefit from individually and even more with a partner or group.

____

____

____

____

Place BEFORE picture here:

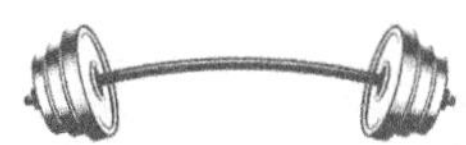

NOW BEGIN **WORKING ON YOUR WELLNESS WISH**

AND ACHIEVE YOUR WOWW!FACTOR!

HOORAY!!!

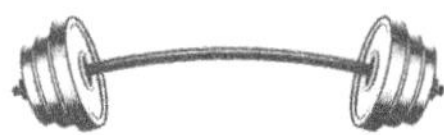

This book is about losing weight and achieving your WOWW!Factor. Remember, WOWW! means Work On your Wellness Wish; and in this case, the primary wellness wish is losing the weight preventing you from living a lifestyle of wellness.

<u>Freedom Key</u>- Set the Stage and Activate WOWW!Factor

1. What would a WOWW!Factor life look like for you?
2. What would you see, hear, experience, etc.?
3. What about your daily habits suggest you are on the right track to achieving your WOWW!Factor?
4. Does your daily routine lead you closer to your goals or father away from it?
5. Are you open to allowing someone help you identify your blind spots? List 2-3 people who could do this for you.
6. Brainstorm what does permanent weight loss mean to you? What does it suggest?

Example:

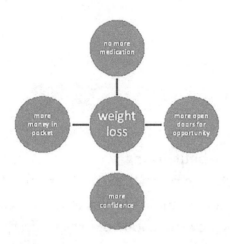

7. What do you believe will be the perks of being fit and healthy INSIDE and OUT?
8. What do you think you will be able to accomplish in this state?

Revisit these questions
as you move throughout the book.

Certain patterns and behaviors lead us AWAY from achieving our WOWW!Factor and living a lifestyle of wellness. The irony is we celebrate and applaud these sabotaging acts because we are grown and no one is going to tell us what to do, especially when it comes to our relationship with food. We get MAD and SAD when the "party in our mouth" ends and reality settles in.

Unclear on what aspect of your life may be **sabotaging** your wellness goals, preventing you from achieving your WOWW!Factor? Keep reading. This book will use the

WOWW!Factor Power Tools of Wellness™ to help you lose physical, mental, emotional, and relational weight and position you for an abundant lifestyle of wellness.

WARNING: If you read and APPLY the concepts in this book and WOWW! yourself, YOU WILL be in the BEST position to successfully lose weight AND KEEP it off.

Total wellness means living in abundance in each of the following areas:

Spirituality	Personal Development
Health/Fitness	Fun/Leisure
Relationships	Finances
Career	Environment

Your level of satisfaction in each area will be based upon the specifics of the season of your life. It may vary from season to season and that is okay. The WOWW!Factor Power Tools can be used to address any area of wellness, but we will target health/fitness or losing weight as the focus of this text, understanding that sustainable weight loss also includes losing mental and emotional weight.

The information is rich and requires *slow digestion*. There will be moments when you may feel like putting the book down or simply give up finishing it. PRESS THROUGH THESE MOMENTS. Pressing through is part of the WORK required to HELP you overcome one of the issues causing you to be overweight. If you must put it down to digest, only do so for a moment. Stick to your reading WORK schedule.

Don't give up*!*

Work On your Wellness Wish!

Place picture of what you visualize <u>after</u> Pic Here

WOWW! FACTOR

LIFESTYLE OF WELLNESS SNAPSHOT

The PERSON who lives a Lifestyle of Wellness ...

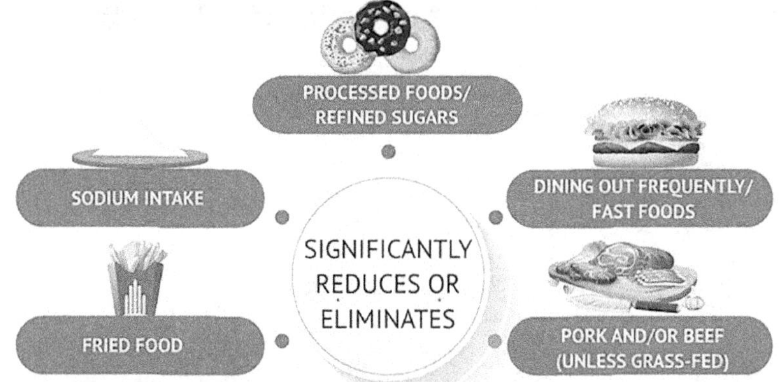

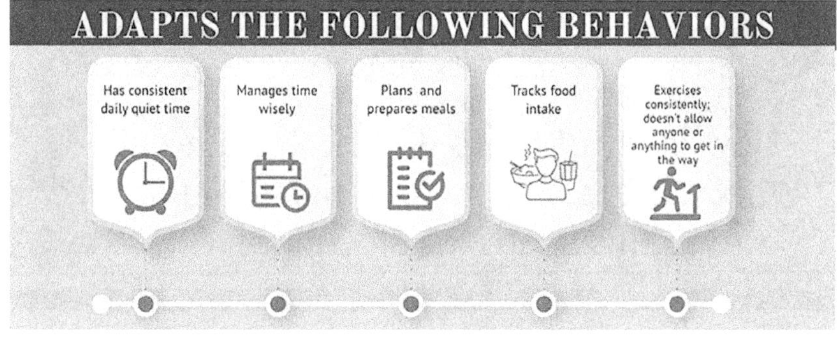

ADAPTS THE FOLLOWING BEHAVIORS
Has consistent daily quiet time
Manages time wisely
Plans and prepares meals
Tracks food intake
Exercises consistently; doesn't allow anyone or anything to get in the way

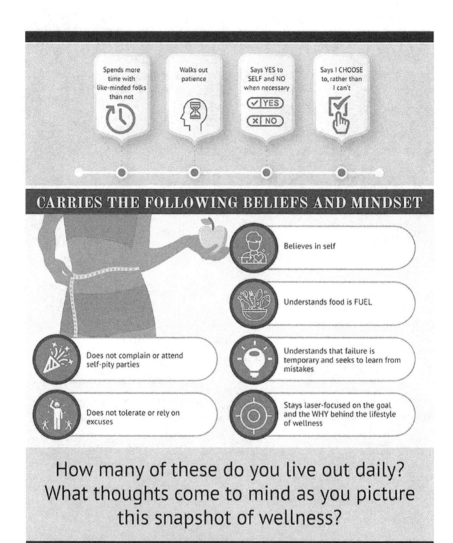
Spends more time with like-minded folks than not
Walks out patience
Says YES to SELF and NO when necessary
YES
NO
Says I CHOOSE to, rather than I can't
CARRIES THE FOLLOWING BELIEFS AND MINDSET
Believes in self
Understands food is FUEL
Does not complain or attend self-pity parties
Understands that failure is temporary and seeks to learn from mistakes
Does not tolerate or rely on excuses
Stays laser-focused on the goal and the WHY behind the lifestyle of wellness
How many of these do you live out daily? What thoughts come to mind as you picture this snapshot of wellness?

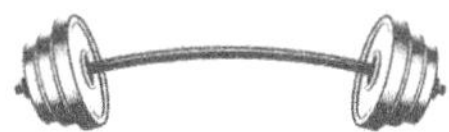

THE STAGES OF CHANGE

Do you want to lose weight temporarily for an event or for the moment, or do you want lose weight permanently? Losing weight and making a lifestyle change towards total wellness are TWO DIFFERENT things that require different pathways.

To identify where you are at today, consider Prochaska and Diclemente's **Stages of Change.**

Pre-contemplation–Change? Change is not for me. I am afraid to change. I will always be this way.
Contemplation–Maybe I can change. Hmmm... My clothes aren't fitting anymore. What are my options? Will it be in my price range? Will I have the time?
Preparation–What do I need to do to change? This program sounds like a good fit. How can I sign up? What do I need to do to prepare and how should I schedule my time? This is an investment in ME!
Action–It's on! I am doing this! I'm changing and not worried about what others think. Exercising and eating healthy is NOT bad at all and I am excited about the slow but STEADY internal AND external results.

Maintenance–I love the new me! I want to stay in this new lifestyle of wellness. I can't meet with you because my workouts are scheduled for this time. Perhaps we can meet on this day at this time? Sunday is my meal prep day and rest day.

Change Reflection Questions

1. When it comes to embracing the tenets of a lifestyle of wellness, which stage of change are you at and why?

____

____

____

____

2. What perceived barriers do you need to address to move to the next stage?

____

____

____

____

To transform your body inside and out, some things MUST change. If you struggle with change, get the assistance of a wellness coach AND continue reading this book.

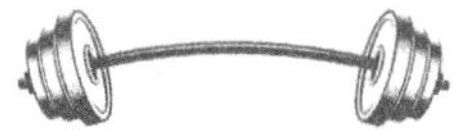

POWER IN PRIORITY

WOWW!Factor PRIORITY Power Tool of Wellness

PRIORITIES—

The *LOUDEST* ___________________ will drive your priorities.

(fill in the blank)

In this lifestyle of wellness, it is imperative that we keep at bay those voices that drive us to not prioritize what it takes to live well.

WOWW! Priority Power Tool–Prioritize and Do HARD things

How about that? Only a few things need to be on your plate at a given time if you want to live a robust lifestyle of wellness. Don't expect others to make YOUR wellness lifestyle a priority for them or even for you. You have to establish it as a priority in speech and action. If you don't, you leave the door open for the priority of others and their desires to take precedence in your life, thus causing your WOWW!Factor to go out the door.

Decide what needs to come to a necessary ending. Who or what needs to be pruned? What people or things are blocking your ability to work on your wellness wishes effectively? When YOU are the priority, you win and so does everyone else as a result of your lifestyle of wellness. Don't believe the lie that you can do it ALL well and accomplish ALL simultaneously.

The cliché is true: if it were that easy, everyone would be doing it. This is where the help of a wellness coach can help you get on the right track. They can help you develop a strategy and implement a plan to do the HARD THINGS until they become second nature. A big challenge for those learning how to live in this wellness lifestyle is making the adjustment to how they view food, scheduling, and priorities. There is often a grief and loss period associated with these areas.

Some people enjoyed the dysfunctional relationship so much with food that the idea of not mindlessly eating can almost send them over the edge. Making time to meal plan and prep and reduce social time or time at the job can send a nervous twitch up one side and back down the other, especially for the extroverts who get their energy from being around others.

The cure: WOWW! with your family and friends or get new friends currently in the wellness lifestyle. Join a fitness group or a wellness coaching cohort. Be okay with reprioritizing your life understanding there is a greater reward on the other side. Some things/people must be pruned for a greater harvest to occur.

WOWW! Priority Power Tool -Time Management

We all only get 24 hours in a day and 7-9 of them should be for sleeping. With the advent of technology, there is a deceptive illusion that we can do more than what we really can and be healthy and fit. NOPE! In fact, many people visibly display they are overbooking their time by the size of their gut. Your gut will often showcase where and how you spend your time and energy. Overweight people tend to be overworked, and often by choice, stress and the corresponding stress eating shows in the belly. Unless you hire a personal assistant, daily chef, daily in-home personal trainer, driver, etc., overworked and overscheduled ruin the recipe for losing weight and living a lifestyle of total wellness.

WELLNESS RED FLAG

Time Management Issues—Allowing time famine to prevent you from doing the hard work.

- WHO tends to get your attention?
- WHAT tends to get your attention?
- WHEN and how often?
- WHAT do they receive from your attention?

- WHAT do YOU receive? Is there an **instant gratification** connection**?**

There is an insidious habit wreaking havoc in your life. It is the one you constantly whisper to yourself—the pass to do IT later.

- I'll do it later.
- I'll eat right later.
- I'll exercise later.
- I'll rest more later.

We do this because it brings a false sense of temporary comfort. It allows us to turn a blind eye to what we need to deal with to move forward. Reality: YOU are in control of your time. You determine who or what gets your time.

Did you know an extreme workload and/or unrealistic schedule can make you fat, especially if it is rooted in fear or the need to please others?

<u>FREEDOM Key</u>— You Only Get 168 Hours Per Week

Determine how much time is currently spent for each activity and write the amount in the ACTUAL TIME column. Determine how much time you need to allow for each activity in order to REDUCE STRESS and still accomplish your top priority goal. Place in the DESIRED TIME column.

ACTIVITY	ACTUAL TIME	DESIRED TIME
Sleep Quiet Time / Devotional		
Exercise		
Meal Planning/Prep		
Church/Spiritual Community*		
Rest/Replenish		
Recreation/Fun		
Family*		
House Management		
Civic Engagement		
Other		
*= circumstantial		

Now that you have a glimpse of WHERE your time is going and where you DESIRE it to go in order to achieve your WOWW!Factor, make the necessary adjustments in your schedule. Set a deadline for implementing the changes. Have your accountability partner assist you with staying on track.

WOWW! Priority Power Tool—Meal Planning and Preparing

Speaking of time management, it is better to schedule a *consistent day to plan and purchase* food, however, many grocery stores offer online grocery shopping with pick-up curbside service. What may normally take an hour out of your day to get in and out of a store can be done in 5 minutes or less with online grocery shopping.

Are you concerned about whether or not they will do a good job with picking out your produce? Relax. They cannot afford to give you subpar produce. They want to keep you as a customer and will do whatever it takes to maintain your satisfaction. Regarding sanitary issues, you should be thoroughly cleaning your produce whether you or someone else put it in your cart.

Save your grocery list (online grocery service automatically saves it) and make modifications as needed. When you are in the lifestyle, you tend to eat the same things on most days because your concern is FUEL and not FUN for your body. You can change up spices and toppings to add variety.

Plan your treat meals or day as well, keeping in mind the focus is not on the party in your mouth but on the FUEL your body needs to meet daily demands.

Unless you like stress, prepare your food in advance for the week or at least half of the week. This will save time and reduce potential stress involved with this part of the wellness lifestyle. If you must have a fresh cooked meal each day all day, more power to you. But if you are like the bulk of us who have a 9-5 job and want to remain fit and trim, we don't have the luxury to desire freshly prepared meals 5 times a day. Food for the daily grind is NOT about an experience, it is about fueling properly to remain fit and healthy.

Identify your designated meal prep day or days. Sundays and Wednesdays tend to work best for most people. If you pick one day, you will need to be prepared to freeze the latter part of the week's meals to prevent the food from spoiling. Get your Tupperware and markers to label measurements and meal numbers to help make the process easier when storing.

WOWW! Priority Tool—Understand Food as Fuel

Understanding the purpose of food is one of the tricks to losing weight and KEEPING it off. Eating healthy choices of whole and minimally processed foods on a daily basis will do wonders for your productivity. Knowing *when* to eat certain macronutrients will help you best utilize them as true fuel sources. For example, eating fruit before bed (just because it is healthy) is unnecessary, especially since it is designed to give you a jolt of energy (great fuel before working out or midday pick me up). Do you really need a jolt of energy right before bed?

Recognize that a relationship with food can be an idol. If food is anything but a fuel source and more like a lover or best friend, you WILL struggle. HOPE is still there, but the work WILL be tougher and the walls that have been erected will take some work to come down. If you have read the Pause and Perspective sections, this should already begin to make sense.

When you understand food as fuel, you stop starving the body. Eating MORE whole foods and nutrient-dense foods will go a long ways to help create feelings of satiety. Whole foods are life-giving, energy- generating fuel foods. Understanding HOW they support the body and not deplete it helps to reduce the over- idealizing of food's purpose in our lives. It is NOT our lover or our best friend; any illusion of that is just that—an illusion.

When you understand food as fuel, you will learn how to manage cravings or at least become more aware of what foods cause cravings and when and what foods do not. Shifting the perspective on food clears space to develop a mind-body connection (an essential of the lifestyle of wellness).

Speaking of mind-body connection, when you have this, you have a better understanding of the message that cravings communicate. Cravings often suggest losing control and are often brought on by stress OR nutrient deficiencies –making it hard to clearly identify what is the REAL need. Don't beat yourself up if you struggle with this. The fact that you are working through this book suggests you are on the right track to a victory in the lifestyle of wellness.

Freedom Key—Need help with understanding your cravings? Join our online WOWW!Factor community at www.wowwfactorwomen.com for additional resources on the topic.

Wellness Red Flag and Freedom Key

Craving	Issue/Potential Nutrient Deficiency	Srategy
Salt/Chips	Stressed/ Sodium, Chloride	Exercise/Fish, Sea salt

When you adopt the mindset of food as fuel, you will:

- Think better.
- Respond differently to potential stressors.
- Have more energy.
- Balance your hormones.
- Position yourself to lose weight.

Have you ever finished creating a great masterpiece after polishing off a plate of fried chicken and waffles with syrup and butter and a side of grits? Probably not. It's a yummy once-in-a-blue moon treat, but this party in the mouth cuisine is certain to do one thing—put you to sleep!

How about coming up with that missing piece to the project after inhaling a double cheeseburger, large fry and an orange soft drink with three little precious Hershey kisses on the side? In most cases creative flow decreases and a feeling of edginess creeps in.

There is science to support what physiologically goes on inside your body as it works overtime to metabolize the party on the palate cuisines. But we will keep it simple for now; we just want to whet your whistle.

The main point is that it's the wrong kind of fuel to consume on a daily basis. Would you put regular gas in a luxury car that requires premium? Of course not; it will affect its overall performance. Your body is a luxury car requiring premium fuel. Say NO to the foods that light the pleasure center of your brain and yes to the foods that help you make money!

In order to continue to use food as fuel, release the Nutrient-Depleters. Nutrient-depleters come in the form of processed foods, sugar and often salt. These are the foods we find in a box or bag on the shelf and/or freezer section of the store. They often contain refined flour and sugar and will often have what we call the white stuff as a main ingredient even if it is disguised as wheat with brown coloring.

Processed foods hijack the body's natural response to whole foods and are energy-depleters. The body has to work harder to metabolize them, slowing the breakdown process for other foods. This rollercoaster of food breakdown leads to insulin spikes and crashes, ultimately contributing to cravings.

Freedom Key—Remove processed foods and sugar out of your system for 7-10 days. Add them back in and note the difference.

About that salt...

The USDA at www.usda.gov recommends 2300 milligrams of sodium intake per day; however, many cannot visibly handle this amount. High sodium intake contributes to bloating and water retention. It also DOES NOT help those suffering from hypertension.

It is NOT a good idea to cut salt altogether as this would be almost virtually impossible to do (even bags of fresh vegetables contain sodium to preserve the product). You don't want your body to become salt sensitive. For those scared to cook with a pinch of salt, pump the breaks. Salt helps preserve food and pull out the bitterness thus drawing out the flavor.

Monitor your sodium intake. Flavor your PREPARED foods with other seasonings; use salt only during the cooking process and use it sparingly.

Limit your dining out experiences. Dining out makes it hard to control exact amount of macronutrient and micronutrient contents i.e. protein, carbs, fat, sugar and sodium. If you find yourself at the local fast-food or eatery more than once a week, then it's time to pause and examine your schedule.

If your schedule demands eating fast food, make sure you have a well-developed plan (preferably laid out with the assistance of a wellness coach) that will allow you to eat the fast food and STILL stay on course. Be willing to consider the Prepared Foods section at the grocery store. This is often "fast" food with many healthy options (and I am not just talking about a measly salad).

Wellness Red Flag—Restaurant foods, even healthy options, contain a lot of sodium for preservatives. Preserving agents are necessary to prolong shelf life of food.

Freedom Key—Fast Food Strategy

Identify 2-3 restaurants where you can get healthy, complete meal options on the run. Looking up menu items in advance is necessary to achieve your WOWW!Factor.

Save the fried foods for the blue moon days. The typical fat content in a serving of fried foods can often be equivalent to 50% of fat allotted for the day. Although we need a certain amount of healthy fats daily, most fried food is not comprised of the good fat. There are several factors that must be considered (weight, height, goal, activity level which all help to determine your overall macronutrient profile), but as a good rule of thumb, keep the fried delights at bay. You will not die without the fried and true.

A word about pork and beef...

Your body needs protein. How much depends upon your body type, goals, etc. Pork and beef have been villainized in the past, but they don't have to be completely off limits for some people. If you are someone who can handle pork or beef, please consider the following:

- Choose the lean, grass fed kind (not pumped up with antibiotics and such).
- These two sources take a longer time to breakdown and LEAVE the body, which is why they are here under the nutrient-depleter category.

WOWW! Priority Tool -Track Food Intake

This one trips many people up. Consider this: Do you keep track of your spending? If you do, you tend to have more success with achieving your financial goals than those who do not. It's not wise to fly by the seat of your pants with spending nor is it wise to do the same with your food. Just like the fuel tank you monitor in your car, you need to track the nutritional fuel you put in your body. Be intentional about what you eat and when you eat so you can clearly identify what is working and you are NOT grabbing for straws in the dark when it comes to losing weight.

There are a variety of apps and online resources to track your food. My favorite online tracking resource is MyFitnessPal at www.myfitnesspal.com. A tracking template is included for those who prefer the old-fashioned paper and pen style.

Up Close and Personal

Calories	Carbs (g)	Fat (g)	Protein (g)	Sodium (mg)	Sugar (g)
1225	190	11	90	3050	80

When looking at the final macronutrient intake totals for the day, one might conclude that this person did well as they only consumed 1225 calories. The problem is the bulk of the calories came from carbs AND the sodium and sugar consumption was high for the day, especially given the sedentary schedule.

To make matters worse, they went UP on the scale instead of down (and did not achieve satiety for most of the day). What happened?

Well, we can only determine what truly happened if we can see a breakdown of food consumption located in the log. Without the log, these numbers only show a glimpse of the obstacle to progress. We need to know which foods were highly processed or from eating out and contributed to the high sodium numbers. What comprised the carbs number? Fruits, starches, candy? How much water was consumed? Tracking thoroughly reduces the amount of wellness sleuthing that needs to take place to make sure you effectively obtain your WOWW!Factor.

Meal	Monday	Tuesday	Wednesday	Thursday	Friday	Satuday	Sunday
1							
2							
3							
4							
5							
Notes							

WOWW! Priority Power Tool–CONSISTENCY

You can consistently do a lot of things right or consistently do a lot of things wrong. Choosing to do what is best to reach your wellness goals and making those choices CONSISTENTLY is what it takes to fully embrace the lifestyle of wellness. If you CONSISTENTLY utilize the tools in this section and book, you are guaranteed to achieve your WOWW!Factor and experience the abundance of a lifestyle of wellness.

In order to make the shift, consider the following:

Passive Approach to Weight Loss AND Cousin to Diet Dumpster Mentality		**Proactive Approach to Weight Loss AND Ownership of the Lifestyle of Wellness**
I've tried that	VS	I CONSISTENTLY do that
I'll try that	VS	I am DOING that

Which column do you find yourself connecting with when it comes to the necessary habits of the lifestyle of wellness?

Are you CONSISENTLY:

- Eating green veggies daily?
- Consuming the proper amount of protein and carbs and fats for your body daily?
- Exercising consistently?
- Resting consistently?

Or are you consistently making poor choices with your health:

- Staying stressed
- Eating poorly
- Not exercising regularly
- Sacrificing rest

BOTH will yield results...

Priority Power Tool Recap—WOWW!

1. In order to WOWW! I MUST make myself a priority.
2. Food is fuel.
3. Consistency is the key for achieving my WOWW!Factor.

STATE Loudly:

I am in the process of consistently doing the "hard" things necessary to achieve my goals.

I am in the process of losing weight and developing a lifestyle of total wellness!

I am working on my wellness wish.

WOWW! I CAN lose weight!

CONGRATULATIONS! You've activated the PRIORITY tool!
Complete the WOWW! Process in journal based upon what you've learned in this section!

WOWW!
Process

What do you need to...

START

STOP

KEEP

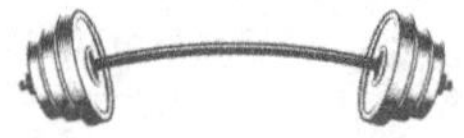

WOWW!FACTOR JOURNAL REFLECTIONS

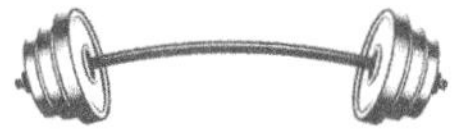

WOWW!FACTOR JOURNAL REFLECTIONS

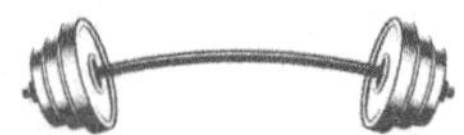

WOWW!FACTOR JOURNAL REFLECTIONS

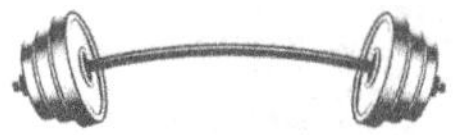

WOWW!FACTOR JOURNAL REFLECTIONS

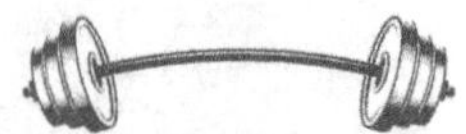

WOWW!FACTOR JOURNAL REFLECTIONS

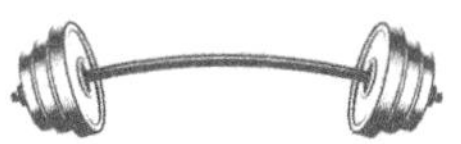

WOWW!FACTOR JOURNAL REFLECTIONS

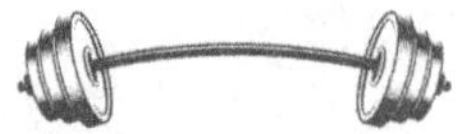

POWER IN PRICE

WOWW!Factor Price Power Tool of Wellness

Invest in Self

Give yourself permission to pay the PRICE necessary to achieve your WOWW!Factor.

WOWW! Price Power Tool- Invest in a New Mindset

Approach the WOWW!Factor process from a growth mindset. Dr. Carol Dweck, in her book *Mindset: The New Psychology of Success*[1], shares the difference between a fixed mindset and a growth mindset. The *fixed mindset* settles that nothing can ever change within a person and offers little room of hope for improvement. Conversely, the *growth mindset* believes there is always room for improvement and with effort and heart, change for the better CAN happen.

<u>FREEDOM KEY</u>—Case Study

Leslie weighed in this morning and gained 2lbs. She later missed her exercise class and opted to stay at work longer to attempt to get ahead. Consequently, she leaves too late to cook dinner and grabs something at a nearby eatery. While waiting on her order, she calls her husband who is preoccupied and doesn't offer much to the conversation.

Response A: I give up. I was meant to be overweight. I should've eaten more food after all. There is never enough time in my schedule. In fact, I just don't have time to lose weight. I've failed at this yet again; I knew it! My husband doesn't support me, and I feel like he wants me to stay this way.

---

1 Dweck, Dr. Carol S. *Mindset: The New Psychology of Success*, (New York, Ballantine Books, 2008).

Response B: Let me review my food journal to see what contributed to the number. How can I plan my schedule next week to make sure I eat on time and exercise consistently? My husband works a lot of hours, so perhaps we can schedule chat/connect time, and I can use my journal to vent and get things off of my chest.

Which one reflects a growth mindset?

Response B reflects a growth mindset. It is the one that gives PERMISSION to look at the situation from a different PERSPECTIVE and opens the door for winning solutions. Embracing a growth mindset will help you own the idea that you CAN Lose weight. Operating with a fixed mindset, will blind you and rob you of the opportunity to win at achieving your WOWW!Factor.

There is a price for releasing a fixed mindset; it's familiar and seemingly safe. It is hard to sacrifice when the return-on-investment is uncertain. However, the real cost and loss comes when you actively CHOOSE to maintain a fixed mindset and remain stuck in a lifestyle that does not reflect the abundance you deserve.

WOWW! Price Power Tool—Change your Wardrobe

Release the clothes of grief (fat clothes or clothes to **hide** in) to clothes of celebration. All clothes, *especially* workout clothes should complement you and have colors that energize you—not matter what your current size is.

Clothes of Grief

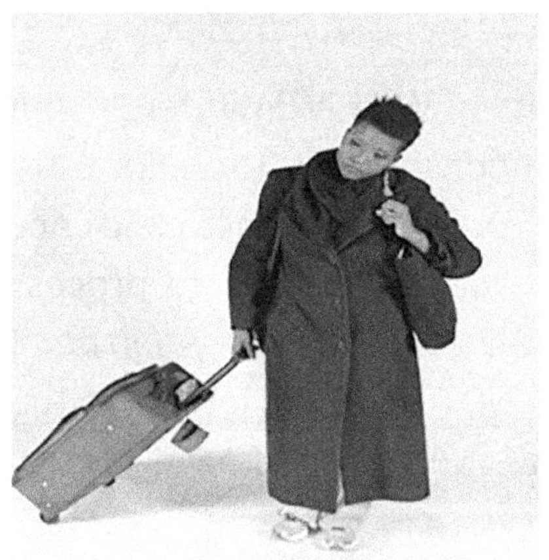

Power Clothes

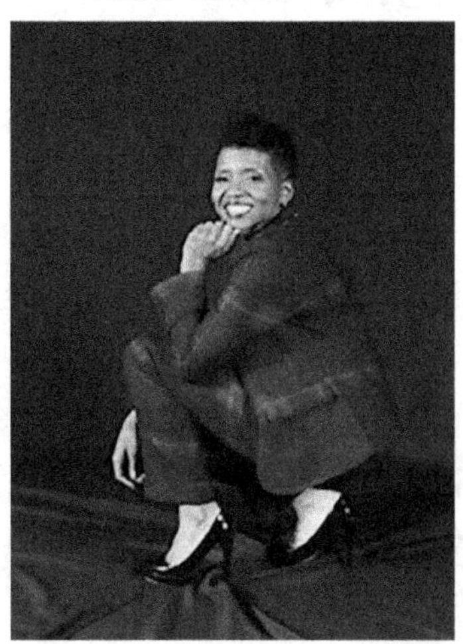

Notice how the clothes of grief come with **baggage.** The baggage reflects carrying unnecessary stress that prevents fully activating the WOWW!Factor.

This doesn't mean you have to go out and buy a bunch of new clothes. Patronize a nice consignment store for attire until you reach the ideal, healthy weight for your body (not the weight that seems easy to obtain). Visit www.wowwfactorwomen.com to get more tips on transitional clothing tips while losing weight.

Here is a secret. When you reach your optimum body weight, you look great in everything—plain clothes, cheap clothes, you name it! Your attitude exudes a lifestyle of wellness and your body physically reflects this truth. As a result, you don't have to work as hard to dress it up. Your confidence will detract from your so-called plain clothes. People are more interested in feasting off the energy and confidence you exude rather than on your wardrobe. But if you are wearing clothes that don't excite you because you want to HIDE your weight, please don't be deceived. It is NOT working, especially for YOU!

WOWW! Price Power Tool—Evaluate Your Environment

Clutter can derail your ability to WOWW! Clutter in your home, on your job, in your relationships, etc., require extra energy that could go towards your WOWW!Factor. Science has proven the brain has to work extra hard to process through clutter even inadvertently. Purge the things you don't need. Purge the things that DO NOT bring you joy. Purge the people who don't bring joy (as much as you have control over that ☺).

Get a system in place that supports the daily habits necessary to achieving your WOWW!Factor (have gym clothes in a bag in car, have a meal prep station in the kitchen, etc.). Use a haberdasher stand to lay out clothes for the next day. Evaluate and organize your environment. Create a space that exudes SUCCESS!

What needs to be in place for you to be successful? What needs to go? Who is and isn't allowed in your environment for this journey? If there are issues out of your control, what needs to happen so they do not erect roadblocks?

WOWW! Price Power Tool—Collaborate with the scale.

There is a price for avoiding the scale. Using how your clothes fit is dangerous deception because you can be 10-15 lbs. up before you need a new size.

Stop villainizing the SCALE. It is an ally, not an enemy. *Don't let the scale bully you*. It is an accountability partner who speaks truth in a short amount of time and in a few words. It sheds light on your habits and schedule but not about the sum total of who you are. It doesn't have the power to label you a *failure* unless you give it permission to do so. It does NOT define you. It may send a love message that it is time to make a change, seek help, tell someone NO, adjust your priorities, and encourage yourself. Kill the lie that the scale is evil.

WOWW! Price Power Tool—Jump IN and WOWW!

Release this notion of "Let me ease into it" or "I need take baby steps" when it comes to losing weight?

DANGER!

It's like saying: **"**please leave the door open so I can return to nonsense and foolishness as I so please," or **"I'm** not really ready to make the commitment yet, but I want to create the illusion that I am" which is self-deception at its finest.

It's very dangerous because after 8 weeks of "easing into it," doing 1/4 of what is required and NOT yielding any real or visible results, discouragement settles in and you quit.

It's simple math: **100% DESIRED results** x **25% effort** = **25% ACTUAL results**. Be nice to yourself and don't expect the tangible benefits of 100% from only 25% of the work required—falling for this is self-torture.

Here are the reasons people choose to *ease* into weight loss?

- An arresting fear of failure

- Grief over the death of old ways *doing* food, exercise, and rest

- Fear of mustering the courage to say NO in order to truly do what it takes

When you start a new job, do you only work 1 day a week and eventually build into a 5-day work schedule *AND* expect a salary like you've been doing 5 days from the beginning? Do you only work 2 hours a day for weeks until you've fully *eased* into 8 hours a day? (With the exception of coming off a traumatic event and easing back into life)

There are times when it makes sense to *ease:*

- Relationships
- Making a major purchase
- Selecting a college to attend
- If you are traveling with Diana Ross and Michael Jackson on the yellow brick road...(couldn't resist)

But once the decision is made and the date is set, *easing ceases*! You jump in and move forward with gotta-get-it gusto! One thing is for certain: Easing into weight loss effort will yield ease on into it results. You cannot get maximum results with ease on into it effort... You deserve better than this!

Hemming and Hawing, Shilly-Shallying, Pussyfooting, Lolly-Gagging, Shucking and Jiving and Piddling around are for birthday agendas and Mother's Day celebrations. These are NOT for people who have made the DECISION to lose weight. There will be NO book on *How to Lose Weight the Shilly-Shally Way* or *The Piddle Off the Pounds Weight Loss Strategy*.

Consider the so-called positives and negatives of maintaining an unhealthy lifestyle (eating choices— eating whatever I want whenever I want, lack of exercise and proper rest, etc.). Doing so should create a sense of urgency and propel you into WOWW!Factor-mode quickly.

<u>Freedom Key</u>— The Con of the Unhealthy Lifestyle

Complete the following chart.

Unhealthy Lifestyle Choice Little to no exercise	**Illusory Positive Benefit**	**Actual Ramification**
Little to no exercise		
Eating whatever and whenever Spending too much time with unhealthy people		

Pay the price, invest in yourself and release the non-productive mindset. Stop the nonproductive behavior that encourages you to *EASE into it* and gives you the **illusion** that you are being productive.

Price Power Tool Recap—WOWW!

1. Release the clothes of grief.
2. Evaluate my environment–create space for success.
3. The scale is an ally for success.

STATE Loudly:

I am in the process of investing in myself and reaping a high ROI!

I am in the process of losing weight and developing a lifestyle of total wellness!

I am working on my wellness wish.

WOWW! I CAN lose weight!

CONGRATULATIONS!

You've activated the PRICE tool! Complete the WOWW! Process in your journal based upon what you've learned in this section!

WOWW! Process

What do you need to...

START

STOP

KEEP

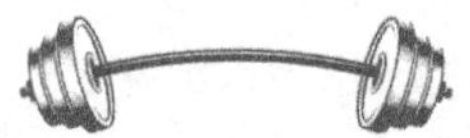

WOWW!FACTOR JOURNAL REFLECTIONS

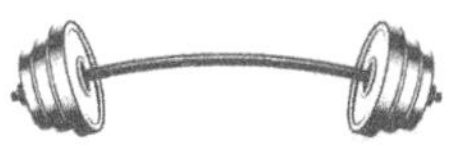

WOWW!FACTOR JOURNAL REFLECTIONS

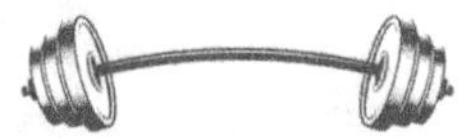

WOWW!FACTOR JOURNAL REFLECTIONS

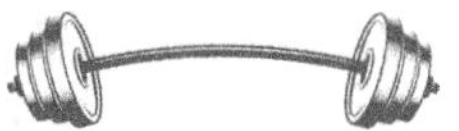

WOWW!FACTOR JOURNAL REFLECTIONS

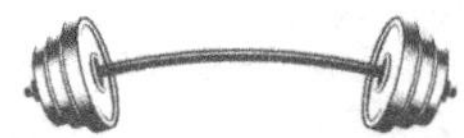

WOWW!FACTOR JOURNAL REFLECTIONS

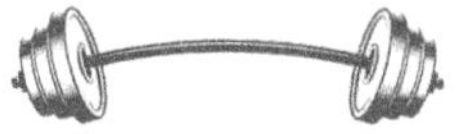

WOWW!FACTOR JOURNAL REFLECTIONS

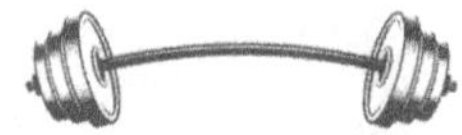

POWER IN PERSPECTIVE

WOWW! PERSPECTIVE Power Tool of Wellness

Your vision determines your success.

If you cannot see yourself as anything but overweight, you will have a tough time doing the necessary work to become fit and healthy as you were designed to be.

You are not created to be unhealthy.
To say you can never be healthy or fit is a lie and one that needs to be cancelled NOW.

Establishing your vision sets the stage to achieve your WOWW!Factor.

WOWW! Perspective Power Tool–TANGIBLE VISION— Imagining the new you is critical for losing weight, getting in shape, and truly embracing the lifestyle of wellness. Once you see it and own it, your brain has created a pathway to do the behaviors necessary to achieve the goal.

FREEDOM KEY—Vision Page Power

Create a vision page with a picture of your head on top of the body you desire. Post it where you can see it daily. Write a vision statement on the page to help make the internal shift. (Sample template provided in *WOWW! I CAN Lose Weight Companion Guide*.)

Up Close and Personal—In order to prepare for a physique competition, I HAD to create a visual of what my body could look like as I consistently trained to grace the stage. Here is an example of my page:

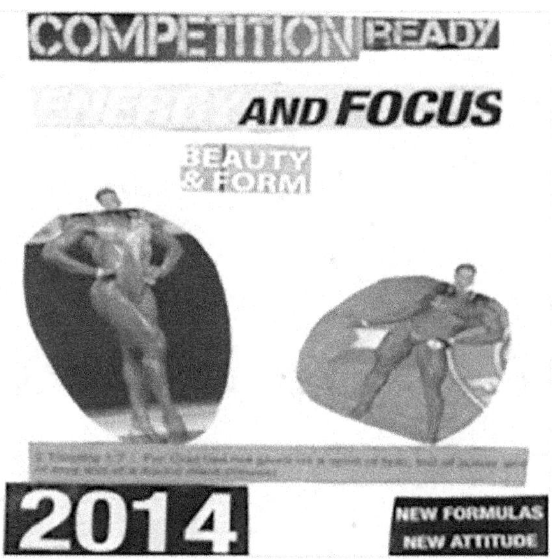

Notice I cut my head off and affixed it to a stage-ready physique. Seeing this daily, especially on training days, helped ensure I made that decisions moved me closer to achieving the vision and fueled me to exercise at the level required to compete.

Having the visual was the first step, but creating a written declaration solidified the process. If you want to SEE something come to pass, writing the vision out is ESSENTIAL!

Up Close and Personal

Here is a sample declaration page that started in a JOURNAL and became a part of my visioning process to achieve my desired goal to compete.

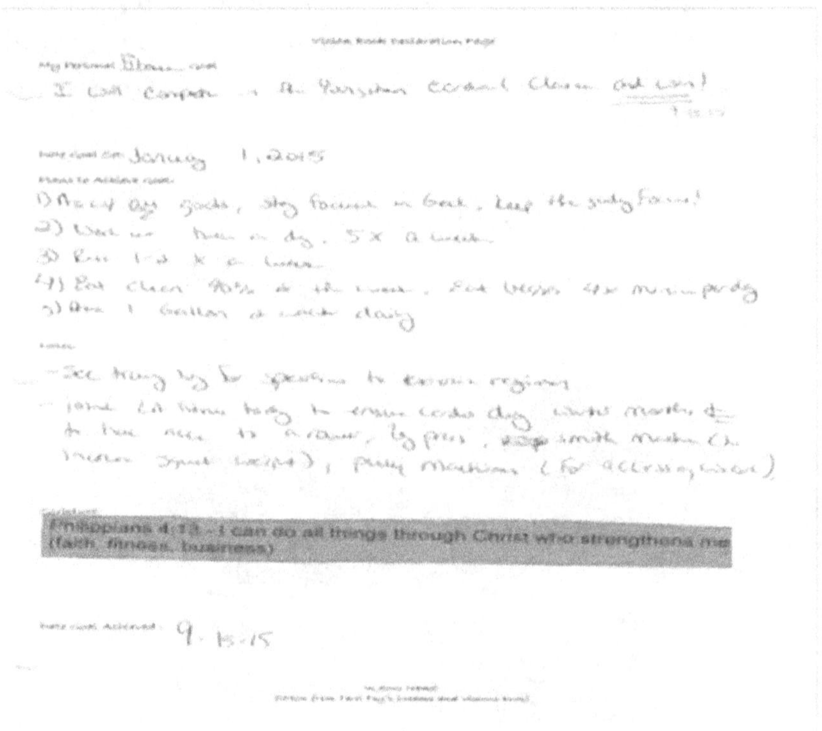

January 1, 2015

Philippians 4:13 - I can do all things through Christ who strengthens me (faith, fitness, business)

9-15-15

(Purchase the ***WOWW! I CAN Lose Weight Companion Guide*** for vision page template and instructions or join the online WOWW!Factor Experience community at www.wowwfactorwomen.com for resources like this and more.)

As you work on shifting your perspective to see a new and healthy version of yourself spiritually, mentally, emotionally, and physically, come to terms with the idea of a new identity fused in with the old. The old you believed certain things about food, exercise, rest, etc.; but, the new you, who embraces the lifestyle of wellness, will courageously believe new truths contrary to the old beliefs. To some degree you *will* seem different even though the healthy parts of you remain the same.

WOWW! Perspective Power Tool-IDENTITY—Establishing a new identity in wellness often creates identity conflict or a *perceived* crisis. With change or transition, we often face conflict at multiple levels and wonder:

a. Am I good enough?
b. Will I be successful?
c. Do I have what it takes?
d. Will people support me?

You are what you believe and will attract THAT which you believe about yourself. If you don't believe you deserve to walk proudly in this new lifestyle and sport all the tangible benefits that come along with it, you will attract people, things and circumstances which will NOT support you. You will find yourself on the merry-go-round of self-doubt and block opportunities for advancement with your name on it.

Wellness Red Flag

You take pride in seeing and STILL NOT believing.

WOWW! Perspective Power Tool—BELIEF SYSTEM— Going through a wellness transformation WILL require a lot of introspection and heavy examination of your belief system. Your belief system is comprised of the thoughts about your life experiences, how you understand them, and the inner vows and bitter root judgments formulated out of these experiences. The messages received from authority figures, family, and peers, such as how to respond to conflict, stress or how to relate to food, will impact your belief system as well.

To better understand HOW your belief system impacts your WOWW!Factor, let's explore your core values. Core values are guiding principles you deem essential and true for living your best life.

What are you core values? Circle your top seven.

Acceptance	Efficiency	Holiness	Rigor
Accountability	Elegance	Honesty	Risk
Achievement	Empathy	Honor	Relationships
Adventure	Dependability	Hope	Relaxation
Awareness	Entertainment	Investing	Reliability
Balance	Enthusiasm	Joy	Rest
Beauty	Faith	Kindness	Simplicity
Clarity	Fame	Modesty	Security
Cleanliness	Family	Nature	Self-Awareness
Collaboration	Flexibility	Obedience	Solitude
Comfort	Freedom	Patience	Speed
Commitment	Excellence	Patriotism	Spirituality
Belonging	Excitement	Peace	Wealth
Community	Exciting	People	Status
Compassion	Generosity	Perfection	Stewardship
Competence	Good Health	Performance	Strength
Competition	Hospitality	Perseverance	Structure
Confidentiality	Humility	Persistence	Success
Conformity	Humor	Personal Development	Support
Connection	Hygiene	Play	Tradition
Consciousness	Imagination	Popularity	Tranquility
Consistency	Justice	Power	Transparency
Cooperation	Leadership	Productivity	Trust
Courage	Learning	Professionalism	Truth
Creativity	Friendship	Profitability	Uniqueness
Discipline	Frugality	Respect	Unity
Diversity	Fun	Progress	Teamwork
Dominance	Hard Work	Prosperity	Winning
Education	Harmony	Prudence	Wisdom
Dedication	Health	Punctuality	Variety
Different	History	Purity	

What are your core beliefs about the following areas and which of your top 7 core values supports these beliefs?

Wellness Area Example: Health/Nutrition	Core Belief I believe food is fuel and not to be used as a part-time lover.	Core Value Connection Discipline Good Health Personal Development
General Health		
Food		
Body Weight		
Exercise		
Finances		
Relationships		
Career		
Family		
Education		
Spirituality		

HOW do you visibly reflect your core beliefs for each wellness category? Give examples for each.

Wellness Area	Actions or Behaviors that Reflect Core Belief
Example: Health/Nutrition	My meals are based upon my activities for the day and fitness and/or general health goals I want to accomplish.
General Health	
Food	
Body Weight	
Exercise	
Finances	
Relationships	
Career	
Family	
Education	
Spirituality	

Distorted Vision is an un-compelling or weak vision which prevents you from moving forward or significantly slows you down. Distorted vision is a result of your belief system. If you struggle with arresting inner vows, bitter root judgments, fear, or doubt, chances are your vision is distorted and preventing you from seeing what's truly possible for you to attain, including living a lifestyle of total wellness.

Distorted vision is created by vision dimmers. A faulty belief system, comprised of vision dimmers, contains **inner vows** and **bitter root judgments**. Dr. Sandy Burkett, in her *Breakthrough Biblical Counseling Course,* defines inner vows as beliefs you hold about yourself formed to protect you from hurt and bitter root judgments are beliefs you hold about others to protect you from harm. [2]

Inner vows, beliefs held about you to protect you from hurt, are often established in childhood from a wound of some kind. If you were teased incessantly as a child for being overweight, you may have formed an inner vow that you will always be fat. Subsequent inner vows may be: "Nothing will ever work for my body to help me lose weight," stemming from the original inner vow that you will always be fat. As a result, all of your actions line up, intentionally and unintentionally, because of the vow erected internally about your body. Fear and Doubt become bedfellows to help keep the vow alive.

Bitter root judgments, beliefs held about others to protect from future harm, are also established in childhood because of a wound from someone else. If you were teased incessantly about your weight by boys, you may have formed a bitter root judgment against men, such as all men are jerks

---

[2] Burkett, Gregg and Dr. Sandy. *Breaking Curses*, (USA, Breakthrough Reconciliation Ministries International, 1987), 35.

or no man will ever see you as attractive. As a result, all of your actions line up with the judgment, thus preventing you from clearly seeing opportunities for men or anyone to help you. Fear and doubt remain bedfellows and help keep the judgment alive.

Wellness Red Flag—Signs of Vision Problems

- **Despondency**
- **Exhaustion**
- **Lack of Mental Clarity**
- **Ongoing Food Cravings**
- **Mental and/or Emotional Numbness**
- **Decreased Motivation**
- **Dysmorphia**

To clear your vision, be mindful of your ear gate and eye gates.

- Ear Gate Activity: What you listen to. What you hear.
- Eye Gate Activity: What you visually take in.

Wellness RED Flag—Watch the ear gate for conflicting messages— half- truths and full lies. Watch the eye gate for the temptation to fall into the comparison syndrome. Lies and comparing yourself with others will certainly mire your ability to see the truth about yourself and compromise your WOWW!Factor.

Your ear and eye gates contribute to how you see the world and how you view a lifestyle of TRUE wellness.

Freedom Key—Ear and Eye Gate Analysis

- What do you audibly and visually digest on a daily basis?
- Does it help you move closer to accomplishing your wellness goals?
- Does it enable you to see yourself as a wonderful creation?
- Does it propel you to walk in a lifestyle of wellness?

Your vision can be strengthened with a consistent employment of the following vision strengtheners:

Surrender—To the idea that you are wonderfully made and are here to fulfill a purpose despite the past hurts and wounds.

Release—The shackles of a faulty belief system and the need to control outcomes and the behaviors of others.

Courage—Face the **truth** (not lies conjured by a faulty belief system) about who you are and activate the courage to do the work to achieve your weight loss goals.

Faith – Have faith in yourself to succeed even when you stumble.

Action—Take action! Work On your Wellness Wish and Win!

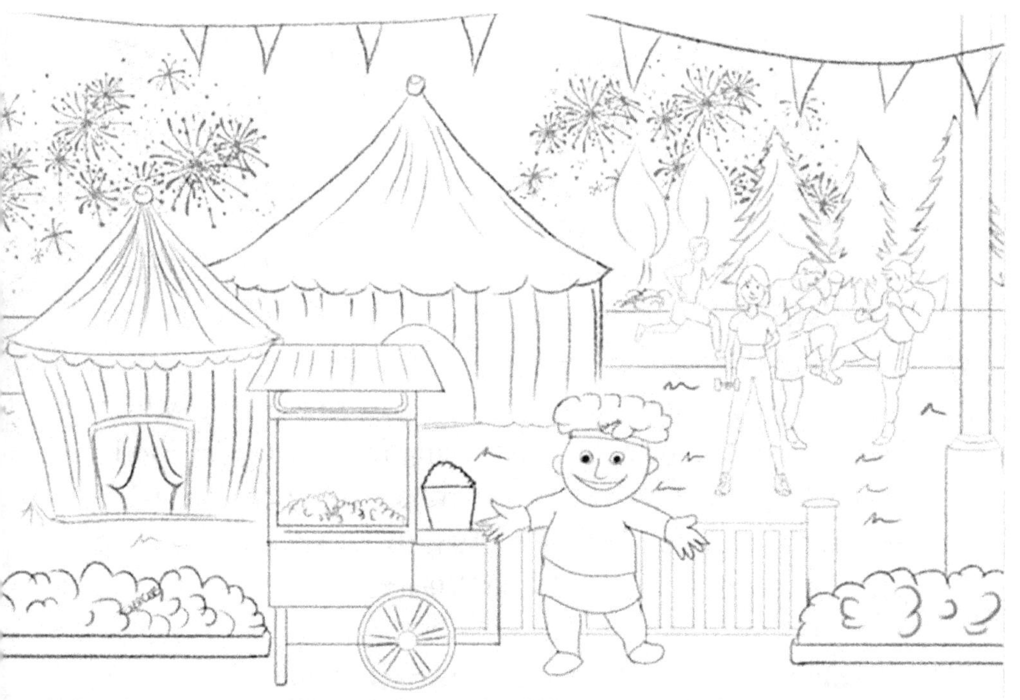

ACTIVITY: Where is your WOWW! Find the WOWW!

a. Where do you begin
b. Where do you look
c. How do you move along the page to discovery—what is the strategy
d. Where do your eyes tend to focus and why
e. What do you tend to gloss over and why
f. Are there any biases or prejudices blinding you
g. Did you become fixated on that which does not matter

h. Was there any vision dimming from your belief system causing you to have blind spots or an inability to see what may be obvious to others?
i. Aside from being a fun, nostalgic experience, what connections can you draw between working through the picture puzzle and going through a WOWW!Factor weight loss experience?

It can be overwhelming and thus easy to give up— which mirrors life and losing weight. Using these WOWW!Factor Power Tools of Wellness™ will help to reduce that overwhelming sensation and clear the way to hear and see what you need to achieve your WOWW!Factor.

Solution: Look right, toward the back , behind the runner, in the grass.

Up Close and Personal—While entertaining a *Where's Mygdaloo* version of this problem-solving experience, I remember being irritated that I had to spend time looking for a dog when I am not a dog lover. What occurred to me was that I was too busy focused on the WHAT to look for in the puzzle and not the WHY behind me pursuing the puzzle in the first place—to successfully solve the puzzle and WIN!

If you have made an inner vow such as "I will always be overweight," OR "I cannot do what it takes to lose weight," cancel the vow NOW and replace it with what is true. You do not have to always be overweight. You CAN lose weight and you have what it takes! People are successfully doing what it takes lose weight and becoming a healthier version of themselves EVERYDAY and the same opportunity IS available to you.

Have the courage to stop acting and thinking like an overweight person. Have the courage to STOP walking out insecurities, unworthiness, dressing with no purpose, living in fear, doubt and shame. Have the courage to stop acting like it is not for you to do WOWW! tasks like planning and preparing your food or exercising consistently. If you think you are fat, you will act fat. If you think you are fit and healthy, you will act fit and healthy and ultimately walk in the wellness lifestyle. "A man always acts according to his thoughts."[3]

If you are overweight and you want things to be different, by faith, start thinking and acting like a fit and in-shape person. You have a choice to act fat or act fit. If you don't know what

[3] Pr. 23:7

this looks like or what thoughts flow from the fit mind, then enlist a wellness coach to help you with level-setting and behavior change. Again, "A man always acts according to his thoughts." Be in the business of renewing the mind DAILY. Use your vision page to help with this process.

What is your vision for this lifestyle? You lose the weight. You are walking out the lifestyle of wellness. What do you see?

Do you just want to lose weight for a second? Do you want to do all the hard work only to go back to old ways which includes gaining weight (and probably then some)? Or, do you want to embrace the hard work as a part of the new normal? Get to a place where you don't think twice about what it takes, you just do it. Keep your exercise appointments. Keep ALL of your wellness appointments. Don't allow ANYONE or ANYTHING to keep you from exercising or doing whatever you need to do to achieve your weight loss goals. Not even the brutal cold weather! Keep the weight off for good! Doing so enables you to experience walking through new doors of opportunity, previously closed to you in the unhealthy lifestyle.

WOWW! Perspective Power Tool- Release the Diet Mentality.

Many people are overweight because they are stuck in a starved situation and only fueling off of nutrient-weak foods often stemming from riding the diet roller coaster over and over. Like a spin on a roller coaster, the thrill is fleeting; it only lasts for a short minute, then reality settles in. I call the mindset associated with dieting "diet dumpster diving" because it requires a lot of unnecessary, unfruitful work that yields precious little, if anything at all.

If you approach your WOWW!Factor with a Diet Dumpster mentality, you will continue to ride the roller coaster of weight gain and loss the rest of your life. If you approach your WOWW!Factor by embracing a lifestyle of wellness mentality, you will not only permanently lose weight, but you will also position yourself to enjoy the process and journey to achieving success.

The following chart illustrates the difference between a diet mentality (i.e. diet dumpster diving) and the lifestyle of wellness:

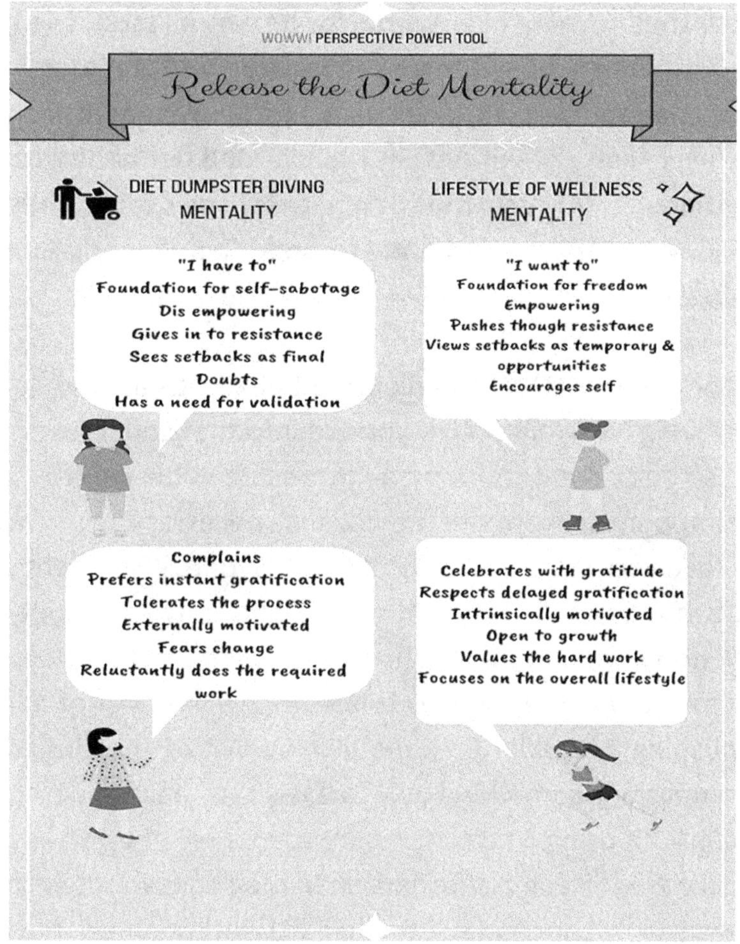

WOWW! PERSPECTIVE POWER TOOL
Release the Diet Mentality
DIET DUMPSTER DIVING MENTALITY
"I have to"
Foundation for self-sabotage
Dis empowering
Gives in to resistance
Sees setbacks as final
Doubts
Has a need for validation
Complains
Prefers instant gratification
Tolerates the process
Externally motivated
Fears change
Reluctantly does the required work
LIFESTYLE OF WELLNESS MENTALITY
"I want to"
Foundation for freedom
Empowering
Pushes though resistance
Views setbacks as temporary & opportunities
Encourages self
Celebrates with gratitude
Respects delayed gratification
Intrinsically motivated
Open to growth
Values the hard work
Focuses on the overall lifestyle

What's interesting about the Dumpster Diet Mentality is that everything can be traced back to some sort of inner vow or bitter root judgment formed in the past. It may not be readily apparent; but, with internal work and EXPECTANCY, it can be revealed. The companion group guide offers more insight on how to identify and address these faulty belief systems that can blur our vision to successfully achieving our WOWW!

<u>Up Close and Personal</u>—Barbara internalized that she doesn't have what it takes to achieve anything and made a vow that nothing ever works for her. As a result, she has to continuously be externally motivated and is reluctant to do the required work because "nothing ever works for her." Her faulty belief system has clouded her ability to see that she CAN accomplish whatever she desires thus blocking the energy and drive to press in and work on her wellness wishes.

The ABSURDITY of the diet mentality is it's akin to dumpster diving for livelihood. If you are into that and it works for you, so be it. But if you want a more sustainable way to make this happen, activate the mental shift necessary.

Have you heard the story of King Sisyphus? His plight was to push a boulder up a mountain DAILY only to have it roll back down again. This was his punishment for deceitfulness.

The irony is that he was forced into a daily act of deceit by pushing a boulder up a mountain creating the illusion of accomplishing something only to have it roll back down again. So it is with using a diet mentality to lose weight and keep it off. Like King Sisyphus, the illusion of moving towards success appears to be the case due to the hard work involved. But like the heavy boulder the king rolled to the top and ultimately rolled back down, you gain the weight back only to have to start the process AGAIN.

This is what the diet mentality does. It keeps you on the roller coaster of gaining and losing until you become frustrated and simply give up and give into the lie that losing weight for good is not your destiny. Thus, you throw your energies into things that yield more immediate gratification. You are done with pushing boulders up a hill only for it to roll back down.

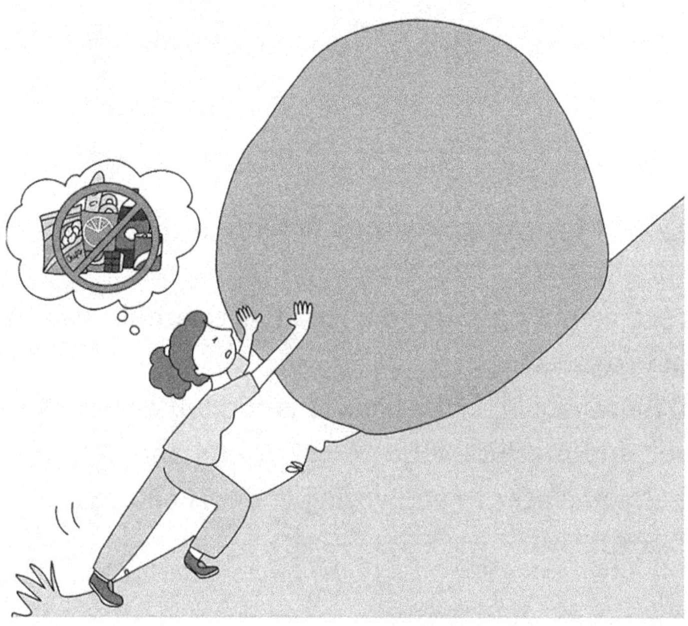

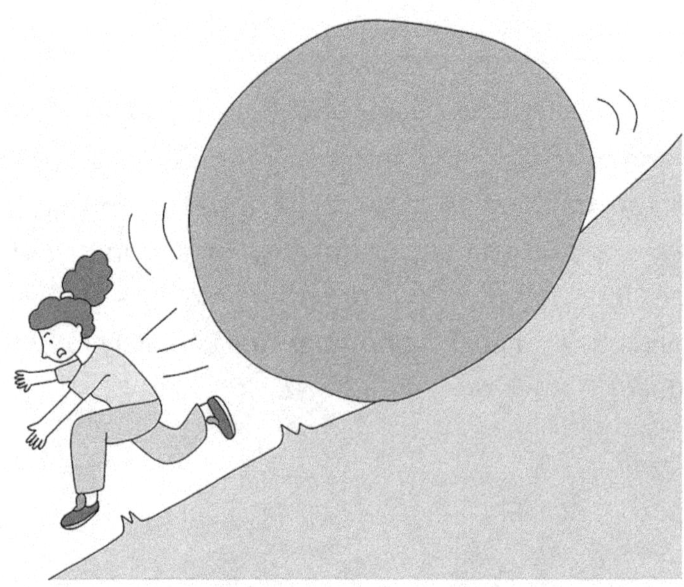

<u>FREEDOM KEY</u>—King Sisyphus Activities

What are your King Sisyphus Activities that only give the illusion of progress?
(HINT: these would be the laborious and futile tasks that wear you out and produce little to no results and definitely DO NOT get you closer to actualizing your vision of wellness for your body.)

____

____

____

____

WELLNESS RED FLAGS

Here are some other deceptive practices and beliefs:

- **Not including EVERYTHING on your meal plan and/or on your tracking sheet**
- **Believing it is okay to put work before exercise**
- **Buying into the illusion that it is okay to sleep only a few hours a day**
- **Pick your daily deception potion____________________**

WOWW! Perspective Shift Power Tool: Recognize Self-Sabotage

Many consciously and subconsciously sabotage their WOWW! when close to achieving success. There is a fear of what will happen if they DO lose the weight. If someone has received negative attention when they were at a normal, healthy weight, there might be a block to going back to that body. The extra weight gives the *illusion* of safety. There is also the fear of still being accepted by peer group when deciding to make WOWW!Factor choices that set you apart. Will they bully or harass me for my daily wellness decisions such as choosing not to participate in the office potluck? Will they ostracize me for preparing my own meal instead? The daunting nature of the unknown can open the door to self-sabotage in achieving your WOWW!Factor.

UP Close and Personal

I have had so many clients say they decided to go off-plan and eat something that did NOT move them closer to achieving their wellness goal because they felt like once they messed up for the day, it was all over. Whenever I hear this rationale for *choosing* to sabotage, I hear someone who is still stuck in a diet mentality that reeks of rewards and punishments. "Since I messed up, I am not deserving of staying on track." "Since I got off course with my exercise, I am not worthy of owning what happened and starting fresh the next hour or next day." When you *Work On your Wellness Wish* and embrace the tenets of the Lifestyle of Wellness, this reward and punishment mindset has no place in your daily living.

To overcome self-sabotage, consider the following:

What do you do when you are the source of your own sorrows? This can be the hardest thing to own when you are the root cause of your frustration. You live with you. You cannot escape you. You cannot divorce yourself when things do not go your way.

When these realities surface, denial sets in. Denial causes you to wear a mask or do things to mask the pain thereby leading to sabotage. Take a *loving* look in the mirror and ask what are you pretending to see? What are you pretending not to see? What are you avoiding? It is hard to accept our responsibility for our mess but vital for perspective- shifting and realignment.

In addition to accepting that YOU led YOU to being overweight, another catalyst for self-sabotage is believing EVERYTHING wellness-related is hard and a major sacrifice.

It may take some initial sacrifices to make changes, but with the proper perspective shift, the sacrifices become just as important as brushing your teeth. When you have surrendered to the tenets of the lifestyle of wellness, you actively leave the old mindset and behaviors behind.

WOWW! Perspective Shift Power Tool—Embrace Delayed Gratification

We inherently have a need to accomplish things. We often lean on things that are EASY to accomplish to gain a quick sense of satisfaction rather than on things that require more work and a delayed sense of fulfillment. Do I dare say we take the path of least resistance?

If we want to feel a sense of euphoria from accomplishment, how does taking the EASY way out really help us arrive at this state? How do we benefit? How do we grow? This false sense of accomplishment derived from the quick fix of instant gratification sets us up for stagnancy and causes us to go backwards in accomplishing our weight loss goals.

<u>Wellness Red Flag</u>—Putting work or career over health.

People tend to put work over health because they can get a quick taste of success or satisfaction. It is easy to fall trap to this because work is familiar and will yield a familiar outcome:

- A paycheck.
- A proverbial pat-on-the-back.

The immediate value seems tangible and easier to actualize than weight loss. The secret irony is: regularly putting your career and/or people over your health diminishes your confidence. It sends a message to SELF that you don't matter and should be treated like you don't matter. If you are willing to treat yourself like you don't matter, this will resonate with others and cause them to intentionally or unintentionally do the same.

It's akin to falling into the entitlement trap. The idea that you can do whatever you want, whenever you want, have as much as you want, and still reach your goals is LIE and a TRAP. When you are committed to eating whatever you want whenever you want and as much as you want and NOT committed to making the necessary adjustments in nutrition, exercise and rest to reach your goal, you have run into an entitlement roadblock to total wellness.

FREEDOM KEY- Use Your Speech to Change Your Perspective

Fill in the blanks:

"_____________________ is actively going through the process
(your name)
to achieve _________________.
(your goal)

What comes to mind as you say this? Journal your response.

Unfortunately, our society has become immune to the idea of delayed gratification; and, consequently, there are a lot of unmet goals and unfulfilled dreams living inside many people.

If you want to fulfill your dream of losing weight permanently, you have to embrace the laws of sowing and reaping (which is grounded in delayed gratification). Since plants do not grow overnight, do not expect a quick fix and immediate weight loss overnight.

- Babies are not created and born in one night.
- You cannot earn a Bachelors, a Masters, or a Ph.D. degree overnight.
- Denzell Washington did not become a star overnight—he was rejected for tons of roles prior to landing the big gig.

Consider lottery winners. Most winners end up worse off than pre-lottery winning. This is often because they didn't go through the ***process*** to EARN the money. Doing the ***Work*** required to earn large sums of money activates the necessary mental shift to *keep* the money and make more. Old belief systems about money built on fear and lack cannot handle a windfall of millions. The old belief system of fear and lack will drive their spending and thus lead them back to zero dollar account balances.

The same is true for weight loss and weight gain.

Harvest is not instantaneous and this is actually GOOD NEWS! A gestational period gives us time to PREPARE to receive the harvest. If you don't know what it's like to walk, talk, and think like a fit person, taking the weight off consistently and at a decent pace will give you a chance to adopt the fit person mindset enabling you to KEEP IT OFF!

WOWW! Perspective Shift Power Tool — Own Your Confidence

The WOWW!Factor requires courage and confidence. I would argue that one begets the other as long as they are exercised regularly. Identify who you have given your power to or where you relinquished your authority. Exercise your courage muscle and take back your power.

Freedom Key — Take Authority!

- Examine WHERE you have given up your authority (Ex: Have you come into agreement that your job owns you and dictates your happiness?)
- What does it look like to have given up your authority or released your power to someone or something?
- Identify what you have authority over.
- Determine what life would be like if you reclaimed that power.
- How will it help you achieve your WOWW!Factor?

Wellness Red Flag—Perfectionism

- **Did you grow up in an environment where it wasn't okay to be perfect?**
- **Are you feeling an oncoming implosion?**
- **Perfectionism is a cousin to laziness as it functions as a means for self-sabotage due to fear of success or fear of failure.**

Perfectionism is a delusional quality that will set you up for failure. Kill the lie that you have to be perfect and that you even are wired to be perfect. As a recovering perfectionist, it takes a daily renewing of the mind to stay delivered from its traps. The WOWW!Factor requires you to take a stand for your wellness and refuse to be bullied by doubt and fear.

Power in Perspective Tool Recap—WOWW!

WOWW!
Process
What do you
need to...
START
STOP
KEEP

1. Maintain a belief system that supports my WOWW!

2. Delayed gratification ensures sustainable weight loss.

3. Fear and doubt will not bully me.

Declaration Activation
STATE Loudly:
I am in the process of releasing the diet mentality and embracing the lifestyle of wellness mindset.

I am in the process of losing weight and developing a lifestyle of total wellness!

I am working on my wellness wish.

WOWW! I CAN lose weight!

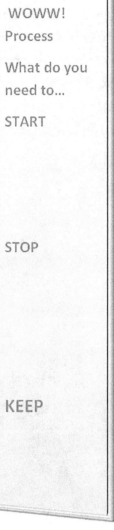

CONGRATULATIONS! You've activated the PERSPECTIVE tool! Complete the WOWW! Process in your journal based upon what you've learned in this section!

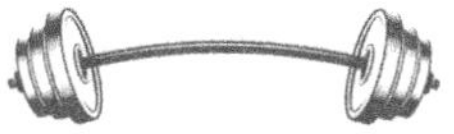

WOWW!FACTOR JOURNAL REFLECTIONS

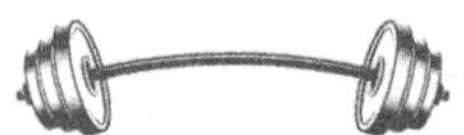

WOWW!FACTOR JOURNAL REFLECTIONS

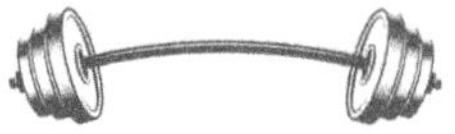

WOWW!FACTOR JOURNAL REFLECTIONS

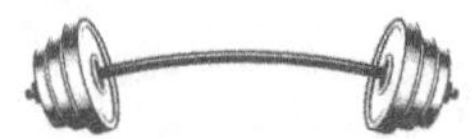

WOWW!FACTOR JOURNAL REFLECTIONS

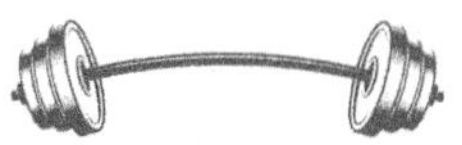

WOWW!FACTOR JOURNAL REFLECTIONS

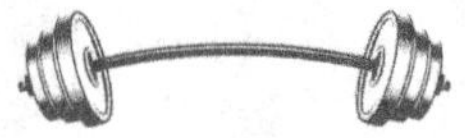

WOWW!FACTOR JOURNAL REFLECTIONS

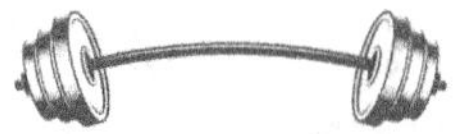

POWER IN PERMISSION

WOWW!Factor Permission Power Tool of Wellness

Sometimes we don't achieve our desires simply because we haven't given ourselves permission to be successful.

WOWW! Permission Power Tool–Embrace failure.

Understand that failure is temporary and an awesome learning opportunity to help you lose weight and keep it off. Shift your mind to seek opportunities to fail; this will enable you to learn and grow stronger. In fact, *release the lie* that it isn't okay to fail and that you must master the entire process perfectly EACH week. The struggle often comes from the erroneous idea that you have to have it all figured out before you begin. Be flexible.

When you fail, do you take full responsibility or do you blame others or look for someone to share the blame for your failure? Don't accept the invitation to throw a self-pity party when you get off course. All invitations are not good. Don't whine or complain. Remember what you speak creates or destroys. Whining or complaining about temporary failure, which is probably only delayed progress, WILL NOT move you forward. Learn from your mistakes and celebrate the progress you WILL make.

Up Close and Personal— I STRIVE to make a mistake daily. It's like cod liver oil, I don't like the taste, but I value what it will do for my body. Mistakes toughen me up and keep me humble. Mistakes are golden opportunities to grow stronger, wiser, and more courageous!

Freedom Key—Mastering Mistakes

Strive to make a mistake daily for the next 7 days. Journal about the experience.

WOWW! Permission Power Tool -Practice Self-Care

Give yourself permission to do the necessary work *DAILY* to replenish and restore your body inside and out. The more you practice self-care, the more likely you will achieve your WOWW!Factor. The more you practice self-care, the more likely you will attract the right people and right things to continue to help you achieve your WOWW! People are naturally drawn to those who look like they invest in themselves.

A snapshot of self-care:

- Sleeping 7-9 hours a day and taking daily moments for mental rest and recuperation. The beauty work happens when the body is at rest. Muscle development, healing and recovery, stress reduction, etc. Depriving your body of rest will certainly be counterproductive in achieving your WOWW!Factor.
- Not falling prey to lies and illusions. *Refuse to believe the lies about your schedule*, the need to please others, that you will never achieve your WOWW!Factor, or that you don't deserve to live a lifestyle of wellness. A lie only takes on life if we breathe on it. The same is true for anything we want to progress or grow. We have to breathe life into it. After all, Adam's life was not activated until God breathed into his nostrils.

Freedom Key—Establishing Your Self-Care

Use the following questions to help you develop a self-care regimen:

- What is your personal rhythm for the day?
- What guidelines are in place to help you stay on target with wellness goals?
- Are your guidelines life-giving or life-blocking?

Permission Power Tool- Spends more time with like-minded folks than not

Ever hear of the crabs in the barrel concept? This is where people, often with good intentions, keep you from progressing because they don't understand what you are trying to do OR it makes them feel uncomfortable or some weird combination of both. If you spend more time with people trying to accomplish what you are trying to accomplish, or spend time with people who are WHERE you want to be, it's more likely you will achieve your goals.

Why? Being around other people in the lifestyle of wellness is a form of accountability. When they make a good choice, you will be more inclined to do the same. When they push hard in the gym, you will be more inclined to do the same. When they make good choices at a restaurant or choose to forgo eating out for an option that lines up with their WOWW!Factor, you will be inspired to do the same.

<u>Freedom Key—</u>Do You Have an Influential WOWW!Factor Circle

Who are the top 5 people in your daily life?

What are their goals and aspirations?

How do they embody the WOWW!Factor?

How do they help you consistently do what you need to Work On your Wellness Wish and embrace the lifestyle of wellness?

How do they hinder you?

<u>Up Close and Personal</u>

One of my clients did the above Freedom Key and realized she was the smallest in her group, thus impairing her ability to see she was overweight and needed to make a change. Compared to her friends, she had it all: the husband, the kids, the house, the career, the income AND she wore a smaller size than all of them, but she actually had an obese BMI which put her in a category for all kinds of health risks. She had to acknowledge the impact her circle of friends was having on her lack of consistency with achieving her WOWW! There was no social impetus to do things differently because the old, unhealthy habits were being validated by her circle of friends.

Be mindful of your social life. Social settings can take you out if you are not vigilante and have not given yourself permission to do WHATEVER needs to be done to safely accomplish your goals. People fear offending others when turning down food offers. Eating with others can often be an unspoken pass for acceptance into a group. We go overkill on the notion that eating builds camaraderie. It can, but it is not the only community builder. There are other ways beyond food to engage in light-hearted activity.

Bottom line, it is OKAY:

- To say NO to situations AND peer pressure that do not line up with the vision for your body.
- To eat your prepared food during the optimum times for YOUR body *despite* how others may feel—it's their issue, not yours. *Don't fall trap to owning problems that DO NOT belong to you.*

Spending more time with like-minded people with similar wellness goals will help minimize potential distractions.

As you monitor your inner circle, be sure to maintain healthy boundaries with everyone. People underestimate how subtle and disruptive peer pressure can be on the journey to a lifestyle of total wellness.

If someone is expecting you to do things for the sake of a project and it requires you to compromise your weight loss goal or general health, ask yourself: Is this person a total reflection of wellness? Even if they are "slim," do they live a lifestyle of miserableness and stress? Are they genuinely and consistently in a state of happiness and peace? Are they fit?

WARNING: Think long and hard before you allow the pressures of someone who DOES NOT reflect total wellness get you off course, especially in the name of a project or some work-related endeavor.

Keep toxic conversations at bay. They are a form of pollution. Would you eat your meals out of the trash? Then why would you ingest polluted thoughts from yourself or others? It DOES have an impact on your WOWW!Factor.

WOWW! Permission Power Tool–NO

People who reflect the WOWW!Factor, value the importance of saying NO and saying YES to self. We understand that most times we do not want to say NO, but we do so for the sake of the ultimate goal. We say NO and keep moving forward with accomplishing our goals.

There is freeing power in the word NO. Sadly, those who find themselves enslaved to the weight often do not have the courage to use this simple yet, mountain moving word—NO.

People have a tough time saying NO:

- To self (when it means abstaining from choices that will not benefit their bodies)
- To people
- To things
- To foods

There are some people, family included, that are not healthy for you to be around during certain seasons. It grieves me to see people burn out trying to reach their wellness goals, with failure looming around the corner. The tough truth is using the word NO more often will lead to progress and satisfaction.

If you have a habit of rescuing people, cancel the agreement it is your responsibility wear the *Red Cape* for others.

Strip the S off of your chest and replace it with NO. Limit the amount of time around folks who play the victim, especially when your rescue efforts interfere with you wellness practices (i.e. exercising, eating right, and resting).

If you know watching TV or taking in certain things at night can impact your ability to get a good night's rest, then DVR for later and say NO to ingesting negativity before bed. This includes negative conversations in the evening. Do you really want the last thing to come out of your mouth or go into your ear before you rest on the pillow to be a conversation about your client, co-worker, or boss who pissed you off? Say NO to the perceived need to process through the negatives of the day before bedtime.

If you struggle with this, there are ways to say no in a way that can soften the blow for the receiver of the NO:

1. Thank you for asking, but I am tapped out at this time.
2. I am unable to commit at this time. Keep me in mind for future opportunities.
3. No, but enjoy yourself. Bring me a souvenir.
4. I have to remain laser-focused this season and do not have the time right now like before.
5. I have to say NO. Why don't you try ___________ (offer a suggestion to consider).

WOWW! Permission Power Tool–Own Truth

Face what you need to face. See what you need to see. Avoidance is not an asset. Shutting down, stonewalling and any other uncooperative behavior will not help you achieve your WOWW!Factor. Remove any self-imposed limitations and shut down the alluring whisper of their lies.

<u>Freedom Key</u>: Conduct a Sincerity Session with Yourself

For your career, relationships, health, and finances respond to the following prompts:

1. List HOW and where you HAVE been truthful.
2. What situations or people do you find yourself avoiding truth?
3. Where is fear driving your thoughts and actions?
4. What are the costs of allowing this fear to rule?

What do you envision once your WOWW!Factor comes into fruition?

Make a choice to STOP saying "I know what to do, I just need to do it." What power is in that statement? NONE. It forces you to remain stagnant at best. It is not an impetus to move forward because it lies to your psyche and feeds your ego, giving you the illusion you "know" something. You fall prey to the deception that you've got it made because at least you "KNOW" what to do. Saying this creates a barrier to getting the proper WOWW!Factor assistance and devising the best strategy to CONSISTENTLY move forward to achieving your goals.

Saying this also suggests you know what to do but don't VALUE enough of what needs to be done or WHY you need to do it. Could it be that you really DON'T know all of what you need to do and the one thing you need is help. Help is not a bad four-letter word.

People often come to our center looking for a weight loss solution but they want the solution to work within the confines of their parameters. What this eventually looks like is people want us to help them lose weight *unrealistically* and often *incorrectly*. If your way worked, you wouldn't be seeking a solution. Either play all in or not at all, understanding that progress does NOT look the same for everyone—(mental progress, physical progress, spiritual progress, emotional progress, visual progress).

<u>FREEDOM KEY</u>—Giving Yourself Permission to WIN

List the top 7 things you need to do to lose weight and KEEP IT OFF.
Rate yourself on a scale of 1-5 with 5 being the highest on how good and consistent you are with doing those things. If your rating is 3 or below for at least 5 of the items, then you need assistance with your WOWW!Factor.

To actualize your WOWW!Factor in your body, some things MUST change. If you struggle with change, get the assistance of a wellness coach. You don't get to keep parts of your counterproductive behavior to blend with your pick of strategies that yield results. Essentially you deceive yourself into believing you don't have to prune bad habits of mind to lose weight. You can't fit a square peg into a triangle hole just because they both have pointed angles.

Stress is the product of having one foot in the old lifestyle and the other in the lifestyle of wellness at the same time. I had a client say this food thing is really stressing them out because they felt like they had to think about food (prep, plan, track) more than they wanted to…when it was really the lie they believed that you can flirt with only certain aspects of weight loss and still experience MAJOR success.

Permission Power Tool
Recap—WOWW!

1. Failure is temporary and a friend.
2. Self-care is essential for WOWW!Factor.
3. Maintaining healthy boundaries is essential.

STATE Loudly:

I am in the process of owning truth and saying NO when necessary to achieve my WOWW!

I am in the process of losing weight and developing a lifestyle of total wellness!

I am working on my wellness wish.

WOWW! I CAN lose weight!

WOWW! Process

What do you need to...

START

STOP

KEEP

CONGRATULATIONS! You've activated the PERMISSION tool! Complete the WOWW! Process in your journal based upon what you've learned in this section!

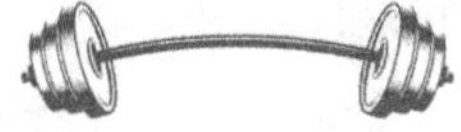

WOWW!FACTOR JOURNAL REFLECTIONS

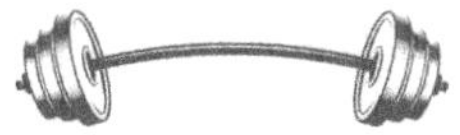

WOWW!FACTOR JOURNAL REFLECTIONS

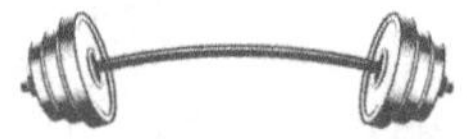

WOWW!FACTOR JOURNAL REFLECTIONS

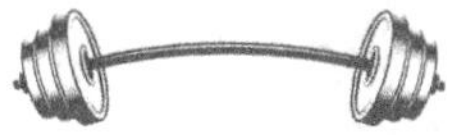

WOWW!FACTOR JOURNAL REFLECTIONS

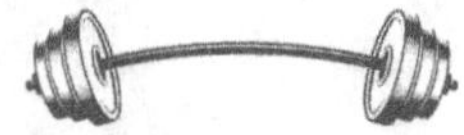

WOWW!FACTOR JOURNAL REFLECTIONS

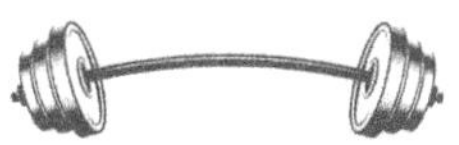

WOWW!FACTOR JOURNAL REFLECTIONS

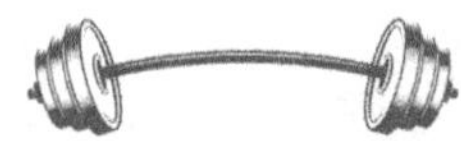

POWER IN PAUSE

WOWW!Factor Pause Power Tool of Wellness

There is power in PAUSE. *Pausing is an essential discipline for a lifestyle of wellness. There are times when pausing is vital before taking the next step to forward to achieving your WOWW!Factor.*

What does it mean to pause?

Pausing suggests:
Being still.
Reflecting.
Breathing.
All of which open the door for
stress and anxiety to dissipate.

Are you taking the time to experience these pause moments daily? If not, the following offers pause tools to help you activate your WOWW!Factor.

WOWW! Pause Power Tool —Quiet Time

Intentional pausing includes a daily regimen of **quiet time**. Many people prefer to start their day with quiet time to center themselves as they prepare for a productive, peaceful day. During this time, some may opt for being intentional about breathing and participate in breathing exercises. In addition to breathing, people may use their quiet time to experience the beauty and simplicity of stillness.

Others opt for ending the day with a pause moment to reflect and release any negativity. Doing this enables the person to learn from the day's experiences and have a better night's rest and positions them for a productive tomorrow.

The key is to pick what works best for you. It could be midday or a combination of ALL three! Depending on what is going on in your life, multiple pauses may be necessary to stay on track for peaceful progress down the road to total wellness.

WOWW! Pause Power Tool-Rest

Rest includes both physical sleep and taking time out from daily activity to restore and replenish your mind and body. In order to successfully lose weight, build muscle or heal from an illness, the body MUST get the appropriate amount of sleep. For the first two, this often means a daily minimum of 7-9 hours of sleep. When fighting an illness, the body will often require more. This is because all of the healing and repair necessary (even from weight training) happens when the body is in a comatose-like state that occurs during sleep. When you are up, there is a certain level of stress taking place just by being up and alert, thereby signaling to the body there is work to be done and this is not the time for recovery.

WOWW! Pause Power Tool —Patience

Pausing creates space to develop PATIENCE. Patience is essential for achieving sustainable weight loss. We often want fast, aggressive returns in lieu of discomfort when it comes to pursuing a weight loss goal, but we must patiently focus on the WHY behind the lifestyle of wellness.

When you commit to and actively walk out patience, you keep the stress monster at bay. Patience is the antithesis of stress. One of our clients reminded us if you are stressed, then YOU are not exercising patience. When it comes to losing weight, be patient with the process. As long as you consistently do the RIGHT things for your body, the weight **will** come off!

What are some of the right things?

- Sleeping at least 7-9 hours per night.
- Eating the right amount of macronutrients (carbohydrates, fats, and protein) and exercising at the right intensity and frequency for **your** goals and body type. This should include weight training.
- Allowing sufficient rest days from exercise per week.
- Drinking the right amount of water for your body and activity level.

Wellness Red Flag—Using coffee to forgo rest? Add an additional 8 oz. of water for every cup of coffee.

Up Close and Personal

There are three main body types: ectomorphs, mesomorphs and endomorphs.

Collete is an ectomorph, who because of narrow frame, fast metabolism and challenge with gaining weight, has to weight train heavier with reps in the 4-8 range and do very little cardio while consuming high density foods with a carbohydrate range being at least 50% of overall nutritional intake in order to gain lean muscle mass.[4]

[4] For more details on body types, join the WOWW!Factor Experience online wellness community at www.wowwfactorwomen.com.

<u>FREEDOM KEYS</u>—Establishing Fruitful Quiet Time

What day of the week can you dedicate (beyond Sunday) to concentrated study time and WHERE?

____

____

____

What time of the day? How much daily quiet time can you devote to replenish? (Ten minutes CONSISTENTLY is better than NO time or sporadic times.)

____

____

____

List THREE ways you will benefit from consistent quiet time.

____

____

____

What potential distractions do you need to be proactive about? What is your strategy?

____

____

____

Pausing helps us recognize when we are genuinely hungry or just using food to feed our emotions. We live in a highly stressed, easily distracted society where the need to pause is crucial to make healthy decisions for our body. Many people gain weight because they use food to ease the stress of the day.

Wellness Red Flag—Buying into the LIE that a lifestyle of stress is normal.

The next time you feel an **emotional eating encounter** occurring, use the HOW to Work through an Emotional Eating Encounter steps to recalibrate and stay on track.

a. Identify WHY you are upset.

b. Identify WHO or WHAT is the source of your frustration.

c. Acknowledge and experience the associated grief.

d. Receive any lessons.

e. Release the stressor (person or event or thing).

f. Keep pressing forward.

g. Celebrate the victory and go do something for YOURSELF — *non-food related.*

You see what just happened here? This was a PAUSE moment to help you get a pulse on what is really going on and discourage you from using food to Band-Aid the issue. PAUSING gives space to own truth and dismiss excuses. Excuses do not make good bedfellows and bully you from achieving your WOWW!Factor.

Wellness Red Flag—Relying on excuses as to WHY you are not achieving your goals instead of owning truth will not help your WOWW!

In his book, *Change Your Trajectory*, Dale Bronner describes an excuse as "a lie disguised as a reason."[5] If you look for an excuse, you will ALWAYS find one.

The following poem explains the fruitlessness of excuses:

Excuses are the tools of incompetence
Used to build monuments of nothingness
And those who specialize in them
Seldom accomplish anything.
Author Unknown

Lose the weight of an excuse.

FREEDOM Key—Pausing and Preventing Episodes of Overeating

Identify patterns that prevent you from being successful and establish new healthy behaviors that create NEW patterns. This will keep you on track with achieving your WOWW!Factor by reducing the default of an excuse.

[5] Bronner, Dale C. *Change Your Trajectory*, (Pennsylvania, Whitaker House, 2015).

1. Identify what day(s) you tend to overeat (all day or specific meals).
2. What time of day?
3. Where are you?
4. Who is with you or who were you just around?
5. What are you doing or what did you just finish doing?
6. What do you tend to overeat? (Probably NOT spinach, asparagus, broccoli etc.)
7. What emotions do you experience right before you overeat?
8. What does the food promise you? What need does food give the illusion it will meet?

WOWW! Pause Power Tool Recap

1. Establishing consistent daily pause moments is essential.
2. Pausing creates space for patience.
3. Pausing positions you to over-come emotional eating.

STATE Loudly:

I am in the process of establishing and enjoying consistent daily pause moments!

I am in the process of losing weight and developing a lifestyle of total wellness!

I am working on my wellness wish!

WOWW! I CAN lose weight!

Congratulations!

You've activated the PAUSE tool! Complete the WOWW! Process in journal based upon what you've learned in this section!

WOWW! Process

What do you need to...

START

STOP

KEEP

WOWW! FACTOR

Actively using the Woww! Factor power tools

Positions you to receive:

1. Favorable treatment from others (right or wrong...but real).

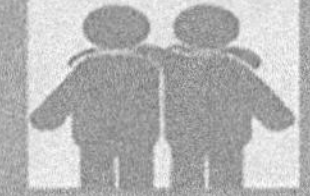

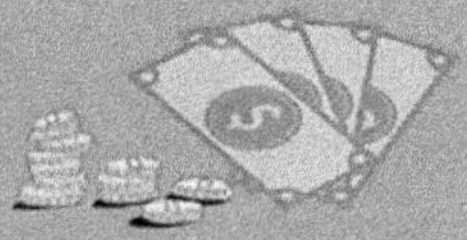

2. More money

3. Better Sleep

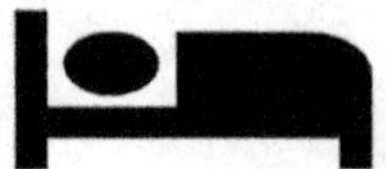

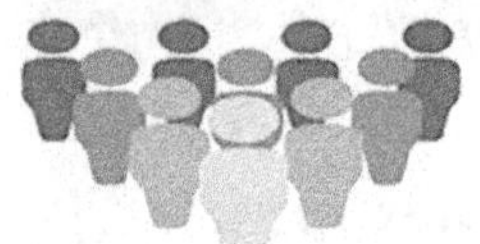

4. Rewarding Relationships

5. Clarity

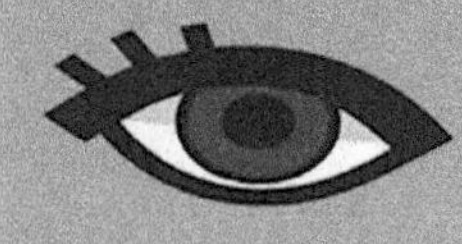

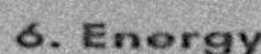

6. Energy

7. More Peace

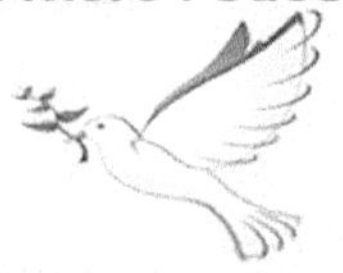

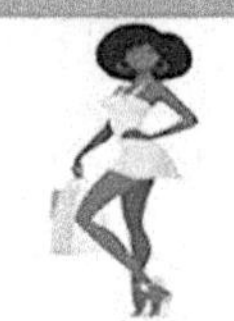

8. Confidence

9. Less Stress

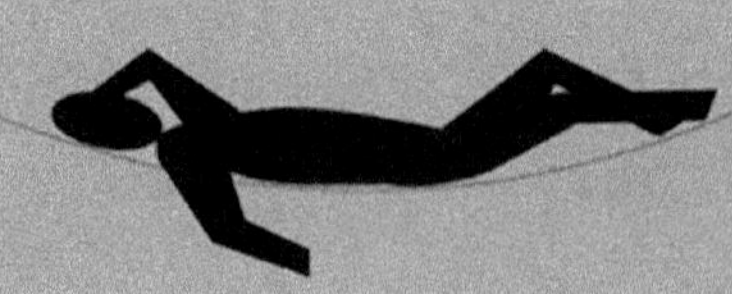

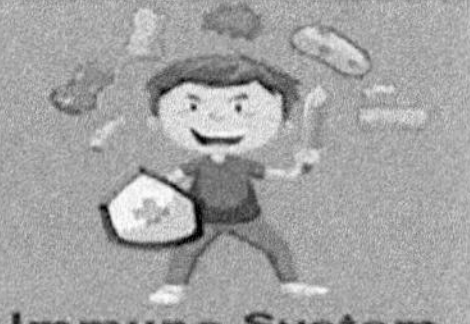

10. Stronger Immune System

11. Simplicity

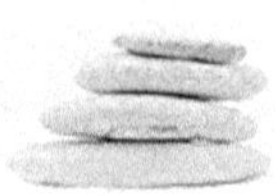

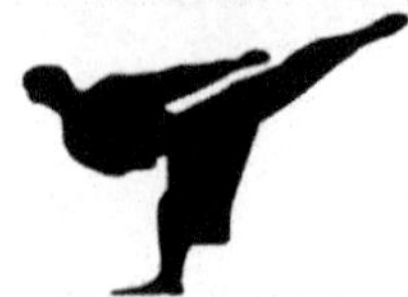

12. Longevity

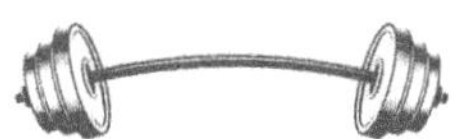

TO ACHIEVE YOUR WOWW!FACTOR

Make YOUR lifestyle of wellness a PRIORITY

Pay the PRICE
Shift your PERSPECTIVE
Give yourself PERMISSION
PAUSING often…
As a part of the PROCESS
And doing whatever it takes **WOWW!** yourself and **WIN!**

Shout: WOWW! I CAN Lose Weight!
Congratulations!

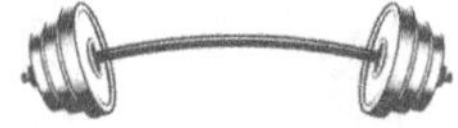

WOWW!FACTOR JOURNAL REFLECTIONS

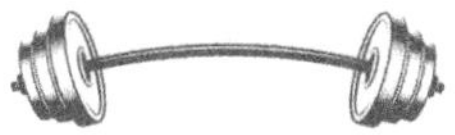

WOWW!FACTOR JOURNAL REFLECTIONS

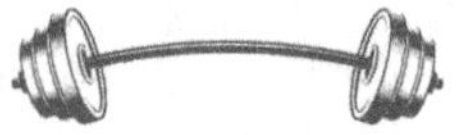

WOWW!FACTOR JOURNAL REFLECTIONS

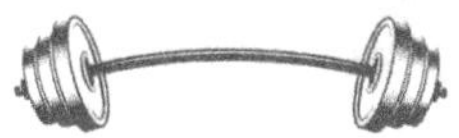

WOWW!FACTOR JOURNAL REFLECTIONS

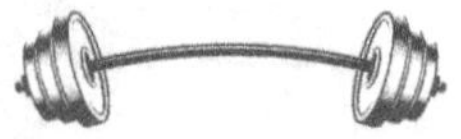

WOWW!FACTOR JOURNAL REFLECTIONS

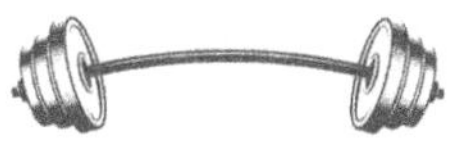

WOWW!FACTOR JOURNAL REFLECTIONS

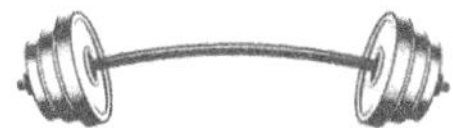

HOW TO ACTIVATE YOUR WOWW!FACTOR

1. Remember the accountability partner(s) you enlisted at the start of the book? Form an official small group dedicated to creating a WOWW!Factor experience.
2. Purchase the *WOWW! I CAN Lose Weight Companion Guide* to help you achieve success.
3. Join the WOWW!Factor online wellness community www.wowwfactorwomen.com. Receive additional WOWW!Factor empowerment tools and opportunities.
4. Believe you can achieve your WOWW!Factor and don't allow anyone or anything to keep you from doing so.
5. Celebrate the pebbles AND the milestones!
6. Love yourself more each day until you love yourself more each day.
7. Subscribe to our WOWW!Factor Experience list www.wowwfactorwomen.com, follow on Instagram and Twitter @WOWW!FactorWoman. Like wowwfactor-woman on FaceBook.

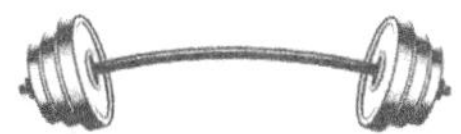

REFERENCES

Bronner, Dale C. *Change Your Trajectory*. Georgia: Whitaker House, 2015.

Burkett, Gregg and Dr. Sandy. *Breakthrough Biblical Counseling Course*. United States: Breakthrough Reconciliation Ministries International, 1987.

Bryant, Cedric, and Daniel Green. *ACE Personal Trainer Manual*, 4th Ed. California: American Council on Exercise, 2010.

Dweck, Dr. Carol S. *Mindset: The New Psychology of Success*. New York: Ballantine Books, 2008.

Fitzgerald, Pia. *WOWW! I Can Lose Weight Companion Guide*. Ohio: Ready Publications, 2019.

Additional Resources to Enjoy

Cloud, Dr. Henry. *Necessary Endings*. New York: Harper Collins, 2010.

Harvey, Steve. *Jump: Take the Leap of Faith to Achieve Your Life of Abundance*. New York: Harper Collins, 2016.

Sanford, John Loren and Paula. *Transforming the Inner Man*. Florida: Charisma House, 2007.

www.wowwfactorwomen.com

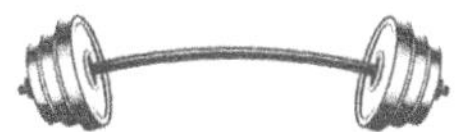

ABOUT THE AUTHOR

Pia Fitzgerald has served in education for over 20 years in a variety of leadership roles while working part-time in the fitness industry. While climbing the career ladder and managing her family, Pia rode the weight loss roller coaster. In 2008, she made the mental, emotional, and spiritual shift necessary to permanently lose weight. Pia happily serves as owner of Baobab Village Wellness Group and Chief Executive Officer of WOWW!Factor weight loss experience. She takes pleasure in helping others implement a transformation plan that moves beyond existence and survival to living life well!

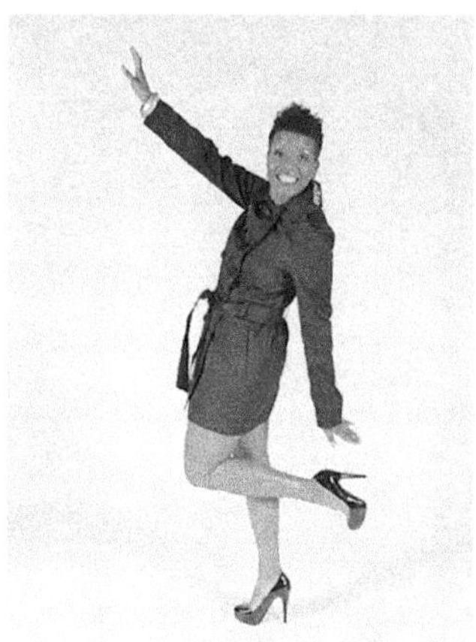

www.wowwfactorwomen.com

CPSIA information can be obtained
at www.ICGtesting.com
Printed in the USA
LVHW022035161019
634412LV00010B/853/P